Silicone Spills

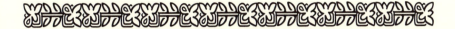

Silicone Spills

Breast Implants on Trial

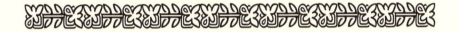

Mary White Stewart

PRAEGER

Westport, Connecticut
London

Library of Congress Cataloging-in-Publication Data

Stewart, Mary White, 1945–
    Silicone spills : breast implants on trial / Mary White Stewart.
      p. cm.
    Includes bibliographical references and index.
    ISBN 0-275-96359-4 (alk. paper)
    1. Breast implants—Complications. 2. Body image in women.
    3. Breast implants—Law and legislation—United States.
    4. Silicones—Toxicology. I. Title.
    RD539.8.S74   1998
    618.1'90592—DC21   97–41006

British Library Cataloguing in Publication Data is available.

Library of Congress Catalog Card Number: 97–41006
ISBN: 0-275-96359-4

First published in 1998

Praeger Publishers, 88 Post Road West, Westport, CT 06881
An imprint of Greenwood Publishing Group, Inc.

Printed in the United States of America

The paper used in this book complies with the
Permanent Paper Standard issued by the National
Information Standards Organization (Z39.48–1984).

10 9 8 7 6 5 4 3 2 1

To My Daughters, Tyler and Kate

Contents

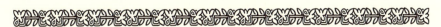

Preface

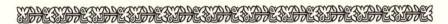

The breast implant debacle is the culmination of factors that alone are troublesome but together are tragic. This story is located at the intersection of corporate greed, the structural inequality of women, and the medicalization of women's bodies. Women, valued for their bodies, yet haunted by their inevitable physical imperfection and decline, are pummeled by endless messages that illustrate their inadequacies and proffer treatments and cures. Constantly vigilant, women turn their focus to reshaping the body, a process in which they are aided by a medical establishment, which has much to gain by expanding its medical turf to include them. Plastic surgeons, working hand in glove with breast implant manufacturers, transform women's natural variations into defects, asserting that there is an objectively acceptable breast and that women who have smaller breasts suffer a disease, which they have the temerity to name micromastia or hypomastia.

Unconcerned by the lack of safety data, plastic surgeons relied on the manufacturers' unwarranted assurances that implants were safe, and placed untested silicone bags into the bodies of hundreds of thousands of women during the past thirty years. Manufacturers relied on the FDA's sluggishness and on their ability to sway politicians and influence policies to keep implants on the market. Even when they had clear evidence that silicone breast implants bled and ruptured, that liquid silicone could migrate throughout the woman's body, and that silicone was not inert but that the human body was likely to develop an immunological response, they persevered.

When the FDA finally responded to women's concerns and complaints about silicone implants and placed a moratorium on their sale in this country, the manufacturers dumped the implants on women in foreign markets, as they had done with the Dalkon Shield.

How could women have been so damaged? How could they have been so dramatically and dangerously failed by the FDA, their doctors, and the corporations that produce medical devices? Is it because women have become so objectified that they are only pieces and parts, breasts and lips and legs, always in need of improvement? Is it because women have been portrayed as receptacles and consumables by men's magazines as well as mainstream films and advertisers? Is it because women have been devalued and discarded as they age, while being encouraged to do endless and hopeless battle with the reality of their changing bodies and faces? Is it because women were already dehumanized that they could be treated like toxic dumps? Is it because women are the display mannequins on which men drape their achievements?

We need to look at this phenomenon from the perspective of the women who, for a plethora of reasons, were willing or eager to get breast implants. But we also need to look at the uglier side of the coin—the faces of those who spent millions of dollars convincing women, doctors, and the FDA that those implants were harmless, with full knowledge that silicone breast implants were potentially devastating both immediately and in the long term. Corporations did not develop breast implants in a vacuum. Rather, they drew upon a culture in which women were eager consumers. Breast implant manufacturers responded aggressively and destructively, unfettered by any moral or legal obligation to consider the toll their negligence would take on women's lives. And now, their efforts are directed at producing "science" that will convince judges to abrogate their responsibilities to take the evidence to a jury of the people. Breast implants have been a tragedy for hundreds of thousands of women. The very corporations that produced this tragedy are now disdainfully devoted to undermining the justice system by evading a trial by jury.

As this book goes to press, Dow Corning Company and attorneys for 400,000 women with breast implants reached a tentative agreement in which Dow Corning offers $3.2 billion to compensate the women in this bitterly contested litigation. The agreement would allow Dow Corning to end its three-year stay in Chapter 11 bankruptcy protection and would compensate women for immune-system illnesses, which they allege are caused by silicone breast implants. It would also provide $5,000 to each woman to have the devices surgically removed. The average amount received by the women would be $30,000, ranging from a low of $5,000 to a high of $250,000 for the sickest women. This settlement is similar to one reached earlier with Bristol-Myers Squibb, Minnesota Mining and

Manufacturing Co., and Baxter International Co. In that settlement, an average of $26,000 was received by each woman. Women still have the option to litigate, but the agreement limits the amounts that would be available. The agreement leaves the dispute about the extent of harm caused by breast implants unresolved.

NOTE

Information on the Dow Corning agreement from Thomas Burton, "Dow Corning implant plaintiffs in accord," *Wall Street Journal*, July 8, 1998, p. A1 and "Implant plaintiffs reach $3.2 billion agreement in bancruptcy action," *Mealy's Litigation Report: Breast Implants* 6, no. 17, July 30, 1998, p. 3.

Acknowledgments

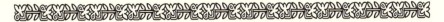

It seems almost a contradiction that an activity requiring so much time in isolation also depends so heavily on others for information, ideas, clarification and support. The women who shared their stories with me made this book possible. They were willing to reveal painful personal experiences to a complete stranger, sometimes opening emotional wounds that had been closed for years, revealing their anger, doubts, strength, and sometimes their physical scars in an effort to have me truly understand their situations and to see them as women rather than only patients or clients. I am also indebted to the attorneys and physicians who spoke with me and who helped me clarify my ideas and who provided documents and insights that would otherwise have not been accessible to me. I am grateful for the fact that courtrooms are public places. I spent many hours observing trials and later interviewing jurors, and was able to develop the context for my analysis of this medical-legal tragedy through those experiences.

There are always particular people without whom the work would have become too burdensome or overwhelming. Jodi Ross, who was my research assistant during much of the data gathering phase of this research, was creative, tireless, and completely reliable. My good friend, Pat Gallagher, gave up precious days of her time to read and reread all of the chapters and to edit and complete the tedious work of compiling the bibliography. Her patient work was indispensable.

Having a well-educated and well-read family has its benefits: Tyler Stewart and Kate Stewart-Hudson, my daughters, Helen Stewart, my mother and my father John A. White, Sr. all helped in different and important ways with the preparation of this book. Cheryl Maes and Laurie Smith, with good spirits and level heads helped with the difficult task of manuscript preparation. Berch Berberoglu, the chairperson of the Sociology Department at the University of Nevada, provided a supportive academic environment that was essential for this work. And, my warm appreciation to Calvin Thomas for his caring and encouragement.

1

Introduction

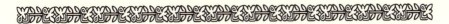

> Dow was aware of possible defects in its implants. . . . Dow knew long-term studies of the implants' safety were needed. . . . Dow concealed this information as well as the negative results of the few short-term laboratory tests performed . . . and Dow continued for several years to market its implants as safe despite this knowledge.
> —U.S. Court of Appeals, Ninth District

During the past three years I have read countless documents and articles, sat through trials, worked with women with implants, interviewed jurors in both federal and district court cases, analyzed questionnaires from women across America, and interviewed many women, talking for hours about their lives and their experiences. All of this, coupled with the gruesome tales about the physical and emotional consequences of implants and the shameless dissembling, maneuvering, and manipulation by defense attorneys, has compelled an exhaustive inquiry of a situation that is not only a complex legal and political controversy but also a personal and social tragedy.

This tragedy is multifaceted. First, of course, is the overwhelming emotional and physical pain suffered by the hundreds of thousands of women who have had silicone gel implants. Fueling this tragedy is the devastating cultural obsession with women's bodies as parts that are never adequate or acceptable, always in need of repair or improvement. Building on this cultural obsession, multibillion dollar multinational corporations manufacture products that have *never* been proven safe nor undergone adequate safety testing for use in women's bodies. When the public, through the efforts of injured women and their attorneys, becomes aware of this negligence, these same corporations mount a multimillion dollar public relations campaign to maintain their position and spend further millions funding studies to manipulate the decisions about the introduction of evidence in court. Furthermore, these same corporations, doggedly devoted to maintaining their political and financial power, lobby tirelessly to destroy the jury system on which justice in this country is based.

The breast implant tragedy has wide-ranging consequences. The corporations' financial and political tentacles have a very long reach: into the offices of plastic surgeons and the boards of medical associations, into the advisory boards of the FDA, into the editorial boards of medical journals, into the epidemiological research conducted by researchers at prestigious universities, into television and print media, and into the courtrooms. These corporations are dedicated not just to protecting themselves from lawsuits by injured women; they are devoted to nothing short of destroying the right of juries to be the deciders of fact in civil cases. They have worked long and hard to convince the public and lawmakers that our courts are overwhelmed with frivolous suits, when in fact there is no such evidence (Huber, 1991; Angell, 1966). Tort suits make up only 9 percent of all state court filings, and product liability suits account for only 4 percent of that (Washburn, 1996). They have worked assiduously to convince the public and lawmakers alike that juries give unconscionably large awards to undeserving plaintiffs. They have labored diligently, under the guise of the neutrality offered by such corporate cheerleaders as Marcia Angell in *Science on Trial* and Peter Huber in *Galileo's Revenge*, to persuade the public and lawmakers that while juries can be trusted to decide whether or not a person is guilty of murder and whether or not that person should go to the gas chamber, they cannot be trusted to make financially consequential decisions about the guilt or innocence of powerful corporations.

The cases of Mariann Hopkins, Charlotte Mahlum, and Maria Stern and Sybil Goldrich are enormously important breast implant cases. They reveal the fearsome, awesome power of everyday people serving on a jury in the United States to punish rich, powerful corporations that are unaccustomed to anyone thwarting their unbridled race for profits. Stunned by these jury awards, which are based on the conclusion that the corporation acted in a "reprehensible" manner, the corporations and their many allies attack the jury primarily on the basis that it cannot be expected to discover the truth amidst the posturing and emotional appeals of slick plaintiff attorneys and as a result will make decisions on the basis of emotion rather than science.

Corporations, then, focus on avoiding the jury completely by convincing the judge that the plaintiff cannot meet the standards for introducing scientific evidence. Specifically, this requires convincing a judge that the methodologies underlying the plaintiff's science are not valid and therefore should prevent the introduction of their research findings to the jury. The defense, on the other hand, pummels the judge with the epidemiological studies, which they have paid for (i.e., Dow Corning gave approximately $8 million to Brigham and Women's Hospital of Harvard University for research to support its defense against claims). These studies are conducted by researchers at prestigious institutions, who also, when necessary, are called upon to serve as defense experts. These studies, they insist, prove that there is no relationship between silicone gel breast implants and the atypical autoimmune diseases that the plaintiffs suffer. These studies prove no such thing, for they are not designed to answer that question. Yet, the public and lawmakers, as a result of the sophisticated efforts of public relations experts, are targeted with this misinformation day after day.

The corporations are making some progress, as indicated by the widely reported Oregon decision by U.S. District Court Judge Robert Jones in *Hall v. Baxter* that affected seventy women in Oregon. The defense was able to keep the evidence from the jury after convincing the judge to grant their motion to exclude and limit the plaintiff's expert testimony. They convinced the judge that the epidemiology showed no association between silicone gel implants and the plaintiffs' illnesses (Kolata, *New York Times*, Dec. 19, 97, p. 1). Judge Jones's wife has breast implants, and that alone should have led him to recuse himself in this case. Barring that, he should have listened to his panel of experts, all but one of whom provided a thorough critique of the methodology rather than an analysis of the research conclusions and indicated that under the *Daubert* evidence rules, the case could be heard. But, as an illustration of a fundamental misunderstanding of the law under *Daubert*, 1993, which establishes judges as "gatekeepers" for the evidence, Judge Jones determined that if the plaintiffs could not prove cause, they could not go to the jury. His ruling, as characterized by defendants, is that "breast implant plaintiffs lack adequate, scientifically valid evidence indicating that silicone breast implants cause any systemic illness, syndrome or autoimmune disorder" (Plaintiffs' Response, 1996:4). The hearing was not to be about cause at all but about whether the methodology of the studies presented by plaintiffs was relevant and valid in light of the *Daubert* mandate to focus on methodology and not conclusions. Judge Jones's action underscores not only the power held by judges in these cases, but also the potential for major corporations to escape the embrace of the justice system in this country by evading a jury trial. This turn of events is potentially devastating. To quote Judge Mark Bernstein in *Blum v. Merrell Dow*, "Castrating the fact-finding role of the jury, the judiciary becomes an absolute bar to legal inquiry, until a new 'scientific consensus' claims the mantle of the divine revelation required to open the courtroom doors, but only to let in the new established orthodoxy" (1996:1027).

The jury system is the bane of huge money interests because it consists of ordinary citizens who cannot be bought and, for this reason, is the very backbone of democracy. The jury system is threatened by these unctuous corporate moves to sidestep traditional justice. In the Mariann Hopkins' case, the jury *was* able to hear the case against corporations, and the jury determined that Dow had acted in wanton disregard for the safety and welfare not only of Mariann Hopkins but also of thousands of other women. The case reveals the importance of requiring that corporations be subject to the jury system on which our entire justice system is built.

Despite my having intimate contact with the women with breast implants, despite hearing about the devastation they experienced and the pain they endured, and despite knowing the frustrations and difficulties associated with their litigation, I could not have anticipated Dow Corning's ugly and outrageously duplicitous appeal of the *Mariann Hopkins* case. Let us look at that appeal from Dow Corning to the Ninth Circuit Court of Appeals in the *Hopkins v. Dow Corning* case (1991).

In 1976, Mariann Hopkins underwent a bilateral subcutaneous mastectomy for severe fibrocystic disease and simultaneously had reconstructive surgery on her breasts, utilizing Dow Corning implants. In 1979, she was diagnosed with mixed connective tissue disease (MCTD). In 1986, as a result of further complications from her breast implants, she had her implants removed and her doctor discovered that they had ruptured. He removed the silicone gel that had escaped but assured her that her ruptured implants could not cause her connective tissue disease. Her ruptured implants were sent to Dow Corning, which found no evidence that any of the damage was related to the manufacture of the implant. Although, by 1987, Hopkins was beginning to believe that her illness could be related to her implants, neither her doctor nor a second doctor she consulted thought any such connection was possible. Finally, on December 1, 1988, Hopkins filed an action against Dow Corning, alleging strict products liability and breach of express and implied warranties.

Evidence presented during the liability phase of the trial showed that Dow rushed development of the implants, creating a Mammary Task Force whose mission it was to get implants to market in less than five months. In its haste to reclaim its position as top producer in the implant market, Dow ignored warnings from its own design team of a "possible gel bleed situation" and refused to make design modifications to reduce leakage. Instead, Dow instructed salespersons to wash the implants with soap and water and "dry with hand towels as the implants become oily after being handled and [bleed] on the velvet in the showcase" (p. 9775). Evidence showed that Dow implants leaked silicone and that they had a high rupture rate. Despite one task force member's suggestion that Dow implement a "double-dip" method as a means of assuring greater uniformity in the envelope, and therefore less likelihood of rupture, Dow stayed with the single-dip method because it was, to use the corporation's terms, "easier" and "cheaper" (*Hopkins v. Dow Corning*, 1991).

The jury also learned that Dow Corning had not conducted research on the long-term effects of silicone implants. For these products which it claimed would last a lifetime, it had done no lifetime studies on animals; the longest study it had conducted lasted only eighty days. In fact, even though this study revealed evidence of inflammatory immune response, Dow Corning continued to market the implants until 1987. Dow had further evidence, which it did not reveal, that silicone was harmful to the human body; after two years, implanted dogs developed inflammation surrounding the implants which demonstrated the existence of an immune reaction. When Dow did reveal this study, it omitted the negative findings and implied that the implants were safe. These were the facts of the case, facts on which Dow Corning was found liable of strict liability, fraud, and breach of warranty. These are the reasons a separate jury awarded Hopkins $840,000 in compensatory damages and $6.5 million in punitive damages.

This is the type of case that leads critics, in their pro-corporation, anti-plaintiff crusades, to condemn the jury system in tort cases, to condemn the plaintiff attorneys who represent injured women, and to call for a ceiling on punitive damages, which they suggest are driving good companies out of business. These are cases, however, one hears over and over in breast implant litigation—cases of enormously profitable multinational corporations, their limitless financial resources and their teams of attorneys, appealing these jury decisions on the basis of objections they established during the trial, not on the basis that they are not guilty or liable for the wrongs the juries found. On what basis did Dow appeal the large punitive damages against it? Did Dow contend that it didn't know silicone was harmful? Did it contend that it did adequate testing? Did it contend that its product did not bleed silicone into the body and rupture easily? No. None of these. Rather, unable to counter the facts on which the jury decided the case, Dow unabashedly appealed on the following bases, acknowledging in its very appeal that it knew early and clearly it was dealing with a product that damaged women.

Dow Corning claimed that the one-year statute of limitations for personal injury claims had expired. Under California law, the statute of limitations begins to run when the plaintiff suspects or should suspect that her injury was caused by wrongdoing. Hopkins testified that she had learned of a possible connection between silicone breast implants and systemic diseases from her mother in December 1987 and filed in December 1988, within the one-year limit. After she became suspicious, she consulted two doctors, both of whom denied any association. Furthermore, her implants had been sent to Dow Corning who reported that the implants "were not defective in any way" (9780). Dow's claim here is shocking. It asserted that when Mariann Hopkins' doctor discovered the ruptured implants, *Hopkins* was responsible for investigating the possibility of wrongdoing at that time. They claimed that because her implants were sent to them for assessment, she was obligated to undertake the investigation of the possibility of wrongdoing. It further stated that a simple investigation by Hopkins would have revealed the possibility of a connection between the implants and mixed connective tissue disease (MCTD), the disorder she had. So, far from denying any wrongdoing or any problems with silicone gel implants, Dow Corning's defense is that she should have "found them out" earlier, and she should have known they were producing a product that could cause connective tissue disorders.

This was Dow's contention, despite the fact that when the implants were sent to them for analysis, Dow Corning assessed them as nondefective. When Dow informed Hopkins of that, it did not mention the possibility of a connection between breast implants and MCTD or other autoimmune diseases. In its appeal, Dow does not defend the safety of its implants, but rather indicates that there were "reports in the published medical literature of suspected immunological sensitization or hyper–immune-system response to silicone mammary implants" (*Hopkins v. Dow*, 1991:9783–9784). Here Dow is basically saying that the implants may well have been unsafe, certainly some research suggested such, and Mariann Hopkins should have found out about it—this despite the fact that Dow never mentioned the possibility. In fact, Dow had taken the position that the product was not defective and she was not injured, and her own doctors saw no connection and were aware of none.

Dow Corning also objected to the court's judgment in allowing the testimony of Hopkins' three expert witnesses. Dow contends that this testimony was not based on scientifically accepted standards. However, the Ninth Circuit found that the *Daubert* decision (discussed in some detail later) upholds Rule 104a and Rule 702, and requires not that the methodologies be generally accepted, nor that the findings be generally accepted, but that the testimony be based on scientific knowledge that will assist the trier of fact (the jury). The Ninth Circuit found that the Hopkins experts based their opinions on scientific methodologies that satisfied requirements established under *Daubert*.

Dow Corning further asserts that it should be exempt from strict liability on the basis of comment K of the Restatement of Torts—that is, it claims that these implants are *unavoidably unsafe*. It makes this claim in its appeal after assuring the physicians, the women, and the public for the last thirty years that silicone breast implants are safe. Dow fought tooth and nail to prevent implants from being classified as a Class III device, requiring safety and efficacy testing, claiming that it should be classified at a much lower level. Then in *Hopkins*, Dow asserted that these implants should be treated the same as prescription drugs and should be seen as "unavoidably dangerous," and thus protected from any liability.

The jury in the *Hopkins* case found that the mammary implant was defectively designed and manufactured, and that Dow failed to warn of a known or knowable risk of harm of the type the plaintiff alleged occurred to her. Under these conditions, Dow could clearly not be exempt from the requirements of strict liability. The damages, which it claimed were excessive, were found by the Ninth Circuit to be reasonable given that thousands of women had been implanted with these devices and were at risk of encountering the same fate that Mariann Hopkins suffered. Dow knowingly exposed thousands of women to a painful and debilitating disease, and it gained financially from its conduct. The company was aware of possible defects in its implants, it knew long-term safety studies were needed, and it concealed from the public negative conclusions from its few studies, continuing to market the implants as safe despite its knowledge. The Appeals Court therefore upheld the punitive damages.

Dow's shameless maneuvering in the *Mariann Hopkins* case was almost unbelievable. Dow, after losing a case in which it asserted that implants were safe and that in fact Hopkins could not be sick from the silicone, appealed on the basis that anyone should have known that implants were unsafe, that it was her duty to see through their lies and deceit and discover that the implants were unsafe, and that furthermore they were unavoidably unsafe and Dow should therefore be protected from lawsuits. One cannot read this case without reeling from the arrogance of Dow Corning, a company that first denied wrongdoing and denied that the plaintiff was sick, and then turned around and contended that of course it was engaged in wrongdoing and she should have known it, and of course she was sick, she had implants that Dow Corning was now insisting were not only unsafe, but *unavoidably* unsafe.

Reading that case was simply devastating. That appeal, more than anything I have read or seen during months of intense involvement with the breast implant controversy, convinced me that Dow Corning and other corporations would stop at nothing to defend themselves against the lawsuits brought by women with implants. This case convinced me that the debate we read in the press, the debate that is of such consequence to the women, takes place on several planes. On one level, there is the effort to present the image that corporations and women simply have an honest difference of opinion about the safety of breast implants, and both sides are eager to discover the truth from the science that is being produced. On the other is the reality that in their brazen efforts to increase profits, the corporations will stop at nothing, whether it is "buying science," lying, deceiving, withholding information, manipulating information, or destroying evidence.

The corporations' efforts to frame the safety issue so narrowly, to construct a reality based on their financial interest, is an effort to manipulate the justice system. Anyone reading *Hopkins*, or watching the Mahlum trial, or reading about Sybil Goldrich knows that the corporations have produced a product that they knew was, at the very least, inadequately tested and potentially dangerous. They are shifting the ground so that the debate becomes reframed as one immersed in the sophisticated, complex interpretations and misinterpretations of scientific theory, methodology, and data.

The basic and most fundamental question, the question on which the breast implant controversy is built, is: "Are silicone gel breast implants safe?" This becomes the most significant question because legal documents and memos uncovered during trial discovery clearly show that companies knew silicone was not inert; knew that implants would leak and bleed; knew that animal studies showed silicone traveling to various organs in the body, including lungs, liver, brain, and kidneys; knew that implants were not adequately tested under sanitary conditions; and knew that women were suffering ruptures and getting sick. The questions now are: what are the consequences of silicone leakage and rupture into the body? Is there a relationship between silicone leakage and the types of nonclassical autoimmune responses seen in women with implants? Can this connection be demonstrated in such a way that Supreme Courts cannot overturn jury verdicts against the manufacturers which are based on a determination that silicone did cause the plaintiff's problems?

The research that is being presented to the public as indicative of the safety of implants is research that does not prove a connection between silicone gel implants and particular classic autoimmune diseases. It does not address the relationship between silicone and atypical autoimmune diseases, nor does it look into the severe local complications that result from implants. The production of science becomes a critical, political issue, and manufacturers are spending millions of dollars to produce studies that they hope will convince judges that the plaintiff does not have enough methodologically sound evidence to the contrary to allow the case to go to the jury. This conflict, which initially involves attorneys and the courts, widens to include the public and the manipulation of public perception. Attorneys for the plaintiffs are waging a battle, with far fewer human and financial resources than the corporations have available, to thwart the corporations' efforts to avoid having the jury decide the facts of the case.

AFTER THE GLOBAL SETTLEMENT

Most of the public thinks that women have at least been financially compensated for the disfigurement and illnesses they have suffered, but that is far from true. In fact, the "global settlement," an agreement for compensation to women with implants reached by attorneys for the manufacturers and the injured women, fell apart after a two-year hiatus during which women were prevented by the conditions of the settlement from bringing suit against corporations if they wanted to participate in the potentially advantageous settlement. It was not until November 1996 that foreign women became eligible to collect any benefits at all. The companies and plaintiffs have been negotiating a possible settlement for women who were in the global settlement (*Lindsey v. Dow Corning Corp., et al.* 1994), since it was dismantled when Dow Corning declared bankruptcy. On August 25, 1997, Dow Corning unilaterally offered to settle legal claims against it with the nearly two hundred thousand women worldwide who have claimed injury and/or illness from implants (*Las Vegas Sun*, August 25, 1997). The $2.4 billion offer was part of a $3.7 billion reorganization plan to recover from Chapter 11 bankruptcy. Claiming that it would "agree to disagree" with the women, Dow Corning offered between $650 and $200,000 to women with varying degrees of illness. In exchange, the women would relinquish their right to make any further claims against Dow Corning or its shareholders.

This offer to settle came a day after Dow Corning suffered a stunning loss in the first class action suit filed against the company. In this case, a state jury in Louisiana found that Dow Chemical had knowingly deceived the 1,800 women in the class by hiding the health risks of silicone used in breast implants and by failing to adequately test silicone before it was used in implants. The jury decision in New Orleans mirrors the verdict in a similar case in Reno, Nevada in 1995, pending before the Nevada Supreme Court. In *Mahlum v. Dow Chemical*, the jury delivered a verdict of $14.2 million against Dow Chemical, including $10 million in punitive damages, finding that Dow Chemical had fraudulently concealed the dangers of silicone from Mahlum.

Dow Chemical continues to assert its innocence. It insists not only that there is no scientific evidence that silicone gel leakage in the body causes autoimmune diseases (as indicated by major epidemiological studies it has funded) but also that if implants do cause disease, Dow Chemical is not responsible since it manufactured the gel, not the implants. It claims not to have been aware that the gel was to be used in implants for the human body, despite the fact that its laboratories were used by its subsidiary, Dow Corning, who manufactured the implants, and despite the fact that Dow Chemical was one of only two shareholders in Dow Corning Company, constituting half of its board of directors.

The fast-paced schedule of litigation proposed for the next two years is situated in a rapidly changing scientific, legal, and cultural context. The recent litigation and settlement negotiations involving states and tobacco companies, the increasing interest in the impact of the *Daubert* decision (discussed in Chapter 9) on the introduction of scientific evidence, and the differential resources available to plaintiffs and defendants in the production of science are among the highly visible issues that shape public understanding of the breast implant controversy. For that understanding to be accurate, any discussion of this issue must acknowledge the impact of power differences, and access to the media and to scientific journals, and the production of science. The discussion that follows provides such a context and acknowledges the attendant contribution of culture and gender to a socio-legal-medical problem that promises to accompany us well into the next century.

During the many years it took the FDA to seriously consider and act in response to the physicians, patients, and scientists who expressed concerns about the safety of breast implants, close to a million women received implants which they, based on manufacturers' representations and plastic surgeons' assurances, believed were safe. Neither the plastic surgeons, the manufacturers, nor the FDA revealed to the public what they knew or suspected about the harm that could result from silicone gel implants (Regush, 1992; U.S. Congress, 1993). However, Dow Corning and other manufacturers, not admitting to the danger of silicone gel implants, did agree to a global settlement under the direction of Judge Sam C. Pointer in Alabama's Northern District. As a result of these negotiations, manufacturers made available $4.2 billion over twenty years to cover damages alleged by approximately four hundred thousand women who agreed to enter the settlement. The settlement was attractive to the women for several reasons: the outcome of a trial is always uncertain, and the women did not have to meet a "Mary Poppins" standard of behavior or lifestyle to receive compensation; the settlement covered future damages and damages to the children of implanted women, and an early settlement would avoid years of waiting for the litigation to end.

During the time this settlement was being negotiated, Dow Corning was already preparing for a Chapter 11 bankruptcy. Court documents indicate that as early as 1993, when Dow Corning entered the global settlement, it was considering a bankruptcy action that would prevent it from being sued and from having to fund the global settlement, thereby protecting its assets. This maneuver, coupled with the two-year hiatus already gained as a result of the extensive settlement negotiations, took place as Congress debated and then passed a tort reform bill that would dramatically reduce the punitive damage awards against corporations found guilty of negligence, wrongful death, and fraud. President Clinton's veto of that bill was understandably met with great joy by the aggrieved implant victims and their attorneys. It was far less welcome news to the manufacturers and corporations.

Some plaintiff attorneys we interviewed suspect that the entire settlement negotiation process was a ruse and an effective stalling technique that resulted in more women dying and thousands becoming too sick, too tired, or too dispirited to continue their legal fight. The women were increasingly powerless, perhaps worn down to the point that they would be willing to take a far inferior settlement to get some compensation and to get the case behind them. The women were exhausted not only by their own symptoms which worsened during this delay, but by the increasingly negative media, the climate in which their credibility was continually challenged, and by the fact that some unprincipled attorneys abandoned them when the global settlement fell apart.

While hundreds of thousands of women were corralled in the global settlement, the corporations were able to fund research, which they could also control, implying that there was no link between silicone implants and the illnesses suffered by these women. Their financial investment and results-oriented interference with the protocols of these studies raise significant concerns about the interface between the standards of admissibility of evidence and the efforts of manufacturers to win lawsuits against them and maintain their market by manufacturing "science" that supports their position. To be unaware of this underlying reality in the breast implant litigation is to forfeit any hope of understanding a tragedy that is sure to plague us for decades.

2

Breast Wishes

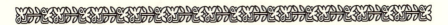

Il faut souffrir pour être belle: One must suffer to be beautiful.
— Anonymous

Karen had silicone implants in 1985 to camouflage a spinal deformity that had long been a source of embarrassment and shame. She initially had considered surgery that involved breaking her ribs and resetting the bones, but a surgeon had suggested that because her breasts were so small and her sternum protruded, breast implants would more success-fully and safely hide the deformity than would a more intrusive opera-tion. She was delighted with that possibility and very satisfied with the results. Her husband, although he had never complained about her body, thought she looked wonderful after the surgery.

She had no problems with her breasts, and felt healthy and strong until her baby was born in 1990, five years after the implants. She didn't seem to bounce back from the pregnancy and birth, and while she tried to attribute her extreme fatigue and fuzziness to postpartum depression, or the effects of the difficulties of labor and birth on her thirty-two-year-old body, she began to suspect something more serious was wrong. Her first thought was of cancer since her aunt and one grandfather had died of cancer. Her visits to the obstetrician following the birth of the baby were normal, and though she listed her complaints, she was eager to agree with her doctor's suggestion that she simply needed to get her mind on something else; nothing was wrong that a little rest and recre-ation wouldn't cure. However, after another four months of increasing fatigue, noticeable forgetfulness, joint and muscle aches, and finding she could barely drag herself through her activities around the house without collapsing, she finally insisted to her doctor that something was seriously wrong. Her clinical exam and her blood tests provided no clues. At about this same time, both her mother and a friend told her about a television show they had seen, "Face to Face with Connie Chung," which aired on December 10, 1990. It was about the problems many women were having as a result of silicone gel-filled breast implants, problems that sounded a lot like hers. But she discounted the similarities and denied the possibility of any connection. She'd been fine until the baby was born, and she loved the way she looked with the implants.

Two more months passed in the same haze and intermittent pain as had the last. She began to see more articles and interviews about implants, and she began to hear about legal cases. She spoke with her doctor, then her lawyer. The lawyer suggested that she see a doctor knowledgeable about diseases related to breast implants to advise her about whether to have them removed; it was, he thought, probable that they were making her sick and that she would not improve until she did. She absolutely refused. After a lifetime of embarrassment about her body, she finally felt normal and could not believe that something like silicone, which she had been told was completely safe, would make her sick. Fortunately, she went back to her own doctor who was now more knowledgeable about autoimmune disease. He suggested different tests and concluded that it was possible that her implants were making her sick. Finally, with great sadness, she made an appointment to have the implants removed. The plastic surgeon, while not agreeing that implants could be her problem, agreed it would be wise to see if they had ruptured.

She scheduled surgery for two weeks later; her husband would be out of town for a few weeks while she healed, and her mother could come take care of the baby. During the surgery, the doctor discovered that both of her implants had ruptured, spilling silicone into her body; her entire chest wall had to be scraped in order to remove the sticky gel from her ribs and tissues. Now, a year later, she is much healthier and stronger, asymptomatic except for some headaches and chronic joint pain. But an ugly scar runs across her entire chest, skin hangs where her breasts were, and her right side is concave. Her spinal deformity is more noticeable than ever. She is convinced that her husband finds her repulsive. Lovemaking takes place infrequently and is restrained because he fears hurting her, or, she thinks, because he has little desire for her.

She had talked to no one about her implants and the damage done by silicone until she agreed to our interview. As we talked over coffee and freshly baked buns in her kitchen, she slowly and cautiously unfolded her story of humiliation and pain. Her delicate coloring and soft voice could not hide her anguish about her body; she felt she had ruined her body by something she had chosen to do, and she understood perfectly why her husband might leave her and begin again. It would have been almost a relief to have that behind her. She had never been to a support group, never shared her situation with a friend. Her shame and humiliation were too great.

Mara and I sat in a back booth at a family restaurant and talked for almost three hours, first about her decision to have implants and later about her overwhelming fear of having them removed. She was young, plain, and very reserved. She was married and had a three-year-old son. Mara's husband worked two jobs now that she couldn't work at all, and she felt terrible about not "pulling her own weight." She was increasingly worried about her ability to care for her toddler and found that the demands, both physical and emotional, were overwhelming her. Although she took an antidepressant, she was so tired and hurt so much that most of the day she lay on the couch trying to entertain her baby with toys and storybooks. She was not only in pain, she was scared. Her body hurt, her head hurt, her breasts were like baseballs, her joints were stiff, her eyes and mouth were dry, she cried "at the drop of a hat." She was afraid she would hurt her baby; she was ashamed of her inability to cook a good meal and clean the house on the same day without collapsing.

Four years earlier, when she was barely eighteen, she had silicone gel implants. After a childhood spent in foster homes, dropping out of high school, feeling ugly and unloved, a man she met encouraged her to become a calendar model but told her she would be much more successful if she had bigger breasts. The plastic surgeon she saw was quick to agree. He stood behind her and cupped her breasts in his hands, inquiring whether she was positive she had never had any children, comforting her with his ability to fix her "snoopy" breasts, and commiserating that no girl her age, who had never had children, "should have breasts like these." She developed a capsular contracture (severe hardening and pain) almost immediately and went back to him complaining of chest numbness, hard breasts, and shooting pains. He performed a "closed capsulotomy"; that is, he pushed her breasts between his hands hard enough to break the scar tissue that had formed in a capsule around her silicone gel breast implants from the chest wall. When she screamed in pain, he responded, "I thought you said you were numb." Mara was frightened. She knew that she must have the implants out but was psychologically frozen, knowing that she would be terribly scarred, that she would be in pain, and that removal would not necessarily remove her symptoms. She hated herself for her cowardice and immobility. After two years of severe illnesses, she had the implants removed. While not perfectly healthy, Mara has more energy, can care for her home and her child, and believes she will continue to improve.

Brenda is forty-six and had a double mastectomy ten years ago. There is a history of breast cancer in her family, and she had lumpy, sometimes painful breasts, a situation eventually diagnosed as fibrocystic disease. After removing several lumps from her breast tissue over several years, her doctor suggested that she have a mastectomy and referred her to a surgeon. The surgeon suggested that because she was so young she would want to have implants to reconstruct her breasts. He assured her that they would never cause any problems, would last a lifetime, and would help her "feel more like a woman." The decision to have the mastectomy was made much easier because of the availability of implants. Seven years later, the fatigue, the muscle and joint pain, the crawling skin sensations, and the headaches were unbearable. Her daughter told her that these problems might be related to her implants. She couldn't believe that would be the case. The surgeon had told her she would go to her grave with the implants; they would last a lifetime, he said. When it was no longer possible for her to go to work, or drive her car because of dizziness and fatigue, or make love because her breasts and body hurt so much, she agreed to see a physician, who convinced her that she should have the implants out. One implant had ruptured, and the other had simply leaked. The surgery was physically devastating because so much silicone had adhered to her muscle and tissue. The plastic surgeon was unable to remove all of it but cleaned out as much as possible, leaving her chest deeply indented and scarred, with uneven flaps of skin puckered and folded where her breasts had been. The headaches and pain and forgetfulness have abated somewhat, but she still has lesions in her brain and silicone in her joints and blood. Her body is constantly geared up for an autoimmune response.

Silicone gel implants are only the most recent in a long history of efforts to increase the size of women's breasts. Breasts have been fashioned as the symbol of women's femininity, the gauge of their womanliness, and women have responded by enhancing their cleavage with everything from makeup to surgery. Many women can remember wearing padded bras or foam "falsies" in their bathing suits, which added inches to the bust but had the unfortunate tendency to slip out and float jauntily on the water when one was swimming. It's the rare woman who can't remember being a teenager stuffing her bra with tissues, even socks, depending on the discrepancy between the reality and the hope, as she dressed for a prom or special date. As adults, women are presented with row after row of lace and satin, cotton and frills on bras that range from slightly padded to almost having a life of their own.

Breasts have been enhanced by bras and corsets of all sorts, flattened by binders, and pushed up, in, and out by various devices. Breasts have always been vulnerable to the changing fashions, these being reflections of the changing expectations for women. Corsets, popular during the period when domesticity, purity, and piety defined femininity, inhibited breathing and movement, allowing for the characteristic frailty, delicacy, and weakness that limited upper-class women to light domestic chores and some quiet leisure activities. Women's bound breasts during the twenties provided a boyish, free, unencumbered look. This style reflected the Flapper Era's allowance that women, at least until they married, had more freedom of movement, a greater ability to act and move in their social world than their mothers had. Later, women's breasts were to be large and full, expressive of the nurturing and protective role women played in the family while their men battled the sterility and alienation of the white-collar world. Women's bodies have been shaped and re-shaped to reflect the roles they play for men in both the family and the workplace—mother, sexual partner, showpiece, child. The body objec-tively displays the woman's identity, and its configuration determines her acceptability and value.

Women's breasts have been injected with substances to enlarge them since the turn of the century. Earlier, a combination of paraffin, petro-leum jelly, and olive oil was used, but silicone injections gained popu-larity during World War II when Japanese women had them to please American servicemen accustomed to larger women with bigger breasts. After the war, during the 1950s, showgirls and dancers, especially in Las Vegas, Nevada, realized that bigger breasts led to bigger paychecks and better roles, and they became the main target for these injections (Byrne, 1996b). By the early 1960s, approximately fifty thousand American women had their breasts injected with liquid silicone. This resulted in enough serious problems and deaths that in 1965 the Food and Drug Administration classified silicone injections as a drug and prohibited them (U.S. Congress, 1993).

Unthwarted by the problems posed by silicone, the search for safer or more acceptable ways to enlarge women's breasts continued, and in 1962 the silicone gel breast implant was developed (Simon, 1995). First used successfully in 1964, implants have now been on the market for almost thirty years with no safety testing, no followup studies (actually, no registry of the women who were implanted was required until 1992 when the FDA severely restricted silicone implants, so it was impossible to accurately track the type and frequency of illnesses in implanted women), and for most of that time, completely unregulated. These devices have been implanted in the bodies of millions of women worldwide without any assurance that they were safe.

Breast implants join Agent Orange, DES, asbestos, Bendectin, and the Dalkon Shield as corporate crimes against the people. Women's bodies are used as experimental dumping grounds for multimillion dollar corporations; they have been used as toxic dumps, and the toxins leaking into their bodies have sickened and sometimes killed them. Corporations have put profits far above the safety and health of women in America and throughout the world.

The powerful voices of women who belong to breast cancer support groups such as Y-ME, which are financially underwritten by the implant manufacturers, as well as the voices of plastic surgeons and the breast implant manufacturers themselves would lead one to assume that most women have implants after mastectomy. Instead, the great majority of women who have implants have them for cosmetic reasons, simply to have prettier, nicer, but especially bigger breasts. Women are capitulating to the demanding entreaties from plastic surgeons, manufacturers, and media to improve themselves through plastic surgery.

Breast implants became popular because of the cultural demands for women to demonstrate femininity in its various forms, the profit motive of manufacturers and plastic surgeons, and the inability of the FDA to protect women in this country from a dangerous product. During the past two decades, an increasing number of women with implants have reported problems ranging from dry mouth and dry vagina to severe headaches, memory loss, cognitive dysfunction, arthritis and rheumatism-like symptoms, extreme fatigue, hair loss, scleroderma, and other symptoms of autoimmune disease. The most frequently cited symptoms are very similar to symptoms of lupus, arthritis, and other rheumatic disorders. Many women have implants that have hardened into tight, painful balls on their chest or that have leaked or bled or ruptured, spilling silicone gel, 90 percent of which is liquid silicone, into their chest cavities. Many have been severely disfigured by the stretching of skin caused by implants or during the effort to remove the silicone from their bodies.

Yet, it was not until April 16, 1992, on the heels of a multimillion dollar jury award against Dow Corning (*Hopkins v. Dow Corning*, 1991) and a subsequent investigation of the FDA's regulation of breast implants as medical devices, that silicone gel breast implants finally were severely restricted by the FDA (Kessler, 1992). Today, manufacturers as well as plastic surgeons, relying on studies largely paid for by Dow Corning, but conducted by researchers at Harvard University and the Mayo Clinic, are calling for the elimination of these restrictions. They claim that there is absolutely no connection between the complaints of implanted women and silicone gel implants.

Manufacturers and plastic surgeons contend that the epidemiological studies remove any concern about the safety of silicone gel breast implants. Indeed, these epidemiological studies (for a variety of reasons that are discussed in some detail later in this book) do not reveal a causal connection between silicone and classic autoimmune diseases, but they certainly do not prove their safety either. The studies have not been sensitive to the atypical illnesses and symptoms the women are experiencing, and are not useful in determining the danger posed by silicone leakage in a woman's body (Simon, 1995; Stewart, 1997). The stories that the women tell speak far more eloquently and cogently to the issue of the safety of silicone gel breast implants, even though they do not represent a random sample of women with implants. Their stories, combined with the history of the development of silicone gel implants and the involvement of corporations in their manufacture, promotion, and distribution, provide the backdrop for understanding the current medical, legal, and social debate about implants and the women who have them.

The debate over breast implants comes during a time when there is vivid interest in so-called junk science, in judicial evaluation of expert testimony, in the role of science in court generally, and in a raging war between corporations and consumers and their attorneys over the issue of tort reform and limits on punitive damages. In an atmosphere heated by litigation and disagreement about the safety of implants and the relationship between choice and responsibility, there are many competing, necessarily self-interested voices: doctors, manufacturers and their attorneys, judges, and, of course, the women and their attorneys.

Some condemn the women as vain and irresponsible for having the implants in the first place. There are also those who assert that women (as men) have a right to do anything they want to their bodies, but they then must take responsibility for these decisions when things go wrong. Many people understand why women have implants, especially after mastectomy, but nevertheless adhere to a "buyer beware" perspective that absolves doctors and manufacturers of responsibility. These evaluations of the choices women make ignore the obvious: that when women were implanted, they were not told of the severe risks of rupture, disfigurement, and disease arising from what they believed were harmless products. Neither are these judgments sensitive to the social and cultural context in which decisions are made. A true understanding of women's desire to enhance their breast size must be situated in an awareness of the everyday realities and strong cultural demands shaping women's decisions about their lives.

Breast implants are hardly the only interventions on women's bodies throughout the world which have been designed to make them salable, acceptable, or valuable. Implants join foot binding and genital mutilation as practices that reflect the willingness to surgically manipulate and deform women in order to make them more aesthetically pleasing to men, thereby making them economically more valuable. Whether the intervention is by an old woman with a piece of glass, an aunt who molds the young girl's foot to make it smaller and cleanses her putrid wounds, or a doctor who slices open her body and inserts a "chemical soup" in a thin plastic bag behind her chest muscle, the underlying reality is the same. Women's bodies are contorted, manipulated, and maimed to conform to a cultural ideal that reflects their economic and political inferiority and their dependence on men for their identity and value.

The women's stories told in this book will help the reader understand the assumptions and expectations that shaped the decision to have implants and that continue to influence their relationship with doctors and lawyers. Their experiences provide a backdrop for the analysis of claims-making in the medical and legal arena, as well as a critique of the impact of economic and social dependence on women's health.

The women interviewed were willing to share their histories and their humiliation and pain. I had the distinct impression that many of them felt that their stories, in whatever form, needed to be told, even if only to me. The opportunity to weave all the threads of their experiences together, was for them healing and validating.

The research process involved talking, listening, and reading medical records, depositions, and transcripts of trials. It also involved understanding the details of work, marital and medical experiences, and the everyday experience of living with either the pain and fatigue of breast implants or the consequences of having them removed. These women spend much of their lives in a "climate of disbelief"; the media, doctors, from general practitioners to neurologists and immunologists, friends, employers, and eventually even family members raise questions about their credibility. Their symptoms were so extensive, so intermittent and diverse, forming such unique constellations, that questions were raised about hypochondria or malingering. Moreover, many of the women are in their forties or fifties, leading many observers to attribute their symptoms of depression, sleeplessness, night sweats, vague pains, and the like to menopause. Many of the women began to question themselves; not a few thought they might be losing their minds, a thought that was not infrequently reinforced by others. It was important to this undertaking that their reality was honored.

The accounts herein, each of them unique, reflect the larger story of breast implants in this country. The story begins with the hundreds of thousands of women in the United States alone, millions more throughout the world who, between 1964 and 1992 decided to have breast implants, usually to augment their breast size or to improve their breast shape. These are the same women who, decades later, are suffering the consequences of silicone bleed and rupture, and who are seeking medical care as well as redress through the legal system in a manufacturer-induced climate of doubt and disbelief. The complex and painful story presented in the chapters that follow is an intricate tale of deceit, malice, and greed, interwoven with culture, gender structure, and the political-ization of medicine. It is a story of the social and economic forces that shaped the damage women suffered as a result of silicone gel breast implants, the pain and destruction of women's bodies and lives, and the legal and medical controversies affecting corporations, plaintiff and defense attorneys, judges and juries, the medical community, and especially the women and their families.

METHODOLOGY

I relied on a wide range of materials in developing this book. I had access to the medical records of over one hundred women who had implants and were involved in the global settlement with manufacturers. These records were extensive, including a very complete description of the women's physical and emotional history, diagnoses, visits to physicians, childbirth and pregnancies, medications and surgeries, and were often accompanied by photos, and sometimes letters from the women. These records also included information about the women's background, such as marital status and occupational history, as well as the entire range of experiences they had with the implants. These records initially served to acquaint me with the medical experiences of the women I was to interview, but more importantly, they also illustrated that recordmaking and recordkeeping only partially reflect the interactions between doctor and patient. Analysis of these records is important because they become powerful tools for both defense and plaintiff during litigation as they attempt to reconstruct the woman's history for a jury.

I conducted in-depth interviews with fifty women who had implants, most of whom were sick or injured. I met them where they would be most comfortable—their homes, a coffee shop, my office. Each interview lasted between one and one-half to two hours. In addition to the historical and social information, much of our interview was open-ended and loosely structured, designed to elicit the subtleties of decision making and reaction to the implants. The interviews were conducted in a conversational style, moving from straightforward demographic information to the more difficult areas of physical consequences of implants and their removal, illnesses, and the impact on relationships with others. The content of these in-depth, open-ended interviews provides the basis for my presentation of the experiences and characteristics of women with breast implants, including their decision-making processes, their reasons for having implants, and their experiences afterward.

To supplement the records and the interviews, I constructed a questionnaire that gathered information similar to what I obtained in the interviews. This questionnaire was lengthy and detailed, including questions about the women's medical and social history, and experiences with implants and with physicians, attorneys, and family. The questionnaires were designed to supplement the in-depth interviews I conducted, and to provide a wider range of information about physical symptoms and such quantifiable information as number of pregnancies, marital status, and other surgeries. Announcements about the research I was conducting were placed in the newsletters of the two largest national breast implant support groups, and women were asked to contact me if they were interested in participating. Sixty-three women from across the country completed and returned the questionnaire. The women who responded are, of course, not a random sample of women with breast implants, nor are they a random sample of women with implants who are involved in litigation, or who are experiencing difficulties. Details of the women's narratives have been changed or combined to assure anonymity while accurately reflecting their experiences.

I did not anticipate the outpouring of pain and misery that I heard from the respondents. Some felt they would die before any settlement could be reached or before any treatment would be discovered, and they wanted to leave a record of their story for other women. One woman did die of lupus, which developed after her Dow Corning implants ruptured inside her chest, spilling silicone into her body. Some were so relieved to have a researcher take them seriously and felt so validated by the interest in their lives that they were eager to complete the questionnaire. Some called, indicating they were too sick to answer immediately, but assured me that they would return the questionnaires as soon as they were strong enough to complete them.

I spent a great deal of time attending support group meetings and listening to the women's discussion of their experiences. Support group meetings often provided an opportunity for women to overcome the isolation they otherwise felt, especially since many had not even told close family members that they had implants. They also provided an opportunity to exchange information about the medical and legal issues with which all of the women were concerned. Again, it is clear that the women's experiences in the support groups are not representative of the experiences of women with implants generally, and I cannot generalize to all women with breast implants.

I also spent weeks in court, as well as pre-trial activities, especially working on *Mahlum v. Dow Chemical* and *Merlin v. 3M*. During this phase, I worked with the clients in preparing for trial, I read depositions, I developed questions to use during *voir dire* (the trial phase during which attorneys and/or judges question potential jurors), and I consulted on jury selection. After the trials, I interviewed jurors in order to discover how well they understood the evidence, the strong and weak points of plaintiff and defense cases, and what they thought of the client and the evidence presented by both sides. I also spent many informal hours with the clients, reviewing depositions and talking about their experiences, gaining insight into their fears and physical realities—all of which provided a backdrop for the responses to more formal questioning.

My participation in a number of other breast implant trials gave me access to these plaintiffs and their history as well as the legal documents accompanying their cases. Much of the information I present in this book about the use of records and the reconstruction of reality results from the weeks spent in court. There I gathered information about medical records and their importance as political documents. In addition, because some of the most important information about a case is provided during the pre-trial hearings, observation of those hearings was crucial in developing the chapter on the impact of evidence standards, in particular, *Daubert*. In addition, I was given access to all of the discovery documents, pleadings, and transcripts that were used during the *Mahlum v. Dow Chemical*, so my access to history is extensive. I have read almost every article, in both the scholarly and lay press, regarding the medical, legal, and scientific aspects of silicone gel breast implants and every article of which I was aware on the history of and controversy surrounding breast implants.

As a researcher, I consciously approached this study from a methodological perspective that placed the researcher and the researched on an equal plane. The women interviewed were not simply subjects, but people with experiences that would help me understand their lives and their decisions. The interview itself was not a one-way question and answer session. Rather, it was a discussion in which the researcher and the researched were on equal ground, sharing information about their lives, especially their personal relationships. This approach to information gathering reflects my assumption that truths and realities are contextual and are constructed from understanding the events in a person's life.

The women whose stories are included in this book are presented not only as clients or patients, but also as mothers, daughters, workers, lovers, and wives. I include here women whose husbands abandoned them when they became ill and those whose husbands have remained supportive and loving through some very rough times. I have talked to women who have implants and are terribly sick, those who no longer have them and yet are still sick, those who have had them removed and are well, and those who have never experienced any problem with their implants. My goal is to elucidate their initial choice, as well as the consequences of the coalition formed by the manufacturers and plastic surgeons, defense attorneys, public relations firms, and medical associations. I trace the politicization of medicine, the creation of a political right and wrong in the area of breast implants, which taints the legal and medical environment in which decisions crucial to these women and the manufacturers are made. I hope to unravel the many tightly woven threads of economy, culture, and politics which make up this controversy.

3

The Path of Destruction: Implant Development, Data Distortion, and the Ineffectiveness of the FDA

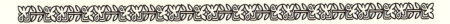

I don't know who is responsible for the decision [to put faulty implants on the market] but it has to rank right up there with the Pinto gas tank.
> —Dow Salesman in a letter to his superior

The manufacturers' plan to keep breast implants on the market without having to demonstrate their safety began to unravel in June of 1988. On that day, the Food and Drug Administration (FDA), belatedly responding to thousands of consumers' and physicians' complaints of rupture, disfigurement, illness, and even death associated with breast implants, ordered the breast implant manufacturers to demonstrate with hard scientific evidence that their products were safe. The manufacturers were unable to demonstrate such safety. Indeed, the scientific evidence that they had successfully concealed from the FDA for so many years demonstrated that the implants were probably unsafe for implantation into animals, much less human breast tissue. After four more years of further government delay, years during which the FDA did virtually nothing to demand responsible behavior from the manufacturers, and during which hundreds of thousands of unsuspecting women underwent surgery to have breast implants, the FDA finally recognized the obvious: not only could the manufacturers *not* demonstrate the safety of implants, but also their scientific research suggested ominous implications for the women who had breast implants.

Finally, on April 16, 1992, the FDA commissioner, Dr. David Kessler, called for severe restrictions on the production and sale of silicone gel breast implants, allowing them only in controlled clinical trials, including women having reconstructive surgery after mastectomy and a limited number of women having breast augmentation (Silverman et al., 1996: 744). This decision was applauded by many, especially sick and deformed women with implants, many physicians who treated these women, and many attorneys who represented the women against the manufacturers. The decision was condemned by others, including implant manufacturers and the American Society of Plastic and Reconstructive Surgeons (ASPRS) who had a substantial financial interest in keeping implants on the market. The manufacturers employed the services of one of the world's largest public relations firms, Burson-Marstellar, and successfully influenced some breast cancer support groups to speak out against the ban.

Kessler's decision was bound to be controversial. But claims by opponents that the FDA acted in haste and before considering all the information were clearly wrong. The FDA's decision came too late as far as many were concerned and only after an investigation by the U.S. House of Representatives Subcommittee on Governmental Affairs under the leadership of Congressman Ted Weiss, (D. New York), which was highly critical of the FDA for its inaction and its comfortable relationship with big business at the consumers' expense. Ignoring or downplaying the urgency of the situation, the FDA had been content to address the concerns of consumers and physicians, as well as reports of dangerous implant leaks and ruptures, through subcommittee and advisory panel reviews, discussion, and recommendations on the safety and efficacy of implants. Unfortunately, these subcommittees and advisory panels were heavily shaped by the financial and political needs of the interest groups involved in producing and using silicone implants.

The FDA's restrictions on silicone gel breast implants were imposed in a climate rife with political posturing. Many conservatives in Congress, following intense lobbying and public relations efforts by various manufacturers, were making every effort to impose ceilings on punitive damages against corporations. The American Medical Association (AMA) and a group of consumers and surgeons calling itself the Citizen's Coalition for Truth in Science (Simon, 1995:151) claimed that the FDA was acting in a paternalistic manner and denying women a voice in their own medical care. Some groups of women with implants, such as Y-ME and the Susan B. Komen Foundation, both of which received funding from Dow Corning (Stauber and Rampton, 1996), insisted that the government was erasing women's choice and denying their freedom. A centerpiece of the manufacturers' public relations plan was a program to convince physicians and reputable medical institutions such as the

AMA and Harvard Medical School to promote the safety of breast implants to the general public. Furthermore, the litigation that helped fuel the FDA's decision, *Hopkins v. Dow Corning Corporation*, revealed that Dow Corning had conveyed false information to consumers about the safety of implants, and that Dow Corning was still refusing to release confidential documents to the FDA. Only after the intervention of the U.S. Justice Department was the FDA able to obtain the relevant "smoking gun" documents from Dow Corning which revealed the extent of its knowledge about the potential danger of silicone gel breast implants.

THE EARLY YEARS: RUSH TO PRODUCTION

What was known about silicone and the safety of silicone gel breast implants prior to the FDA's restriction of their availability? Prior to the development of implants, beginning in the early 1950s liquid silicone had been used to augment breast size. This silicone fluid was industrial grade silicone, transformer coolant, mixed with cottonseed oil or olive oil to cause immediate scarring, in order to contain most of the gel at the site of the injection (Simon, 1995). Soon, plastic surgeons and other doctors in Nevada and California were injecting silicone between the pectoral muscles of the chest wall and the back of the mammary tissues of exotic dancers and show girls, a technique known as the Sakurai formula after the Japanese doctor who originated it. The results were disastrous; many women suffered gangrene, pneumonia, and massive infections. Women who received the injections also suffered such complications as granulomatous hepatitis, hypopigmentation, blindness, fevers, elevated liver enzyme levels, and sometimes, death. Studies on injected silicone reconfirmed fears of catastrophic systemic effects. The silicone sometimes migrated to other parts of the body, accumulating in lumps in the neck, arms, or chest. Removal of these lumps often could not be accomplished without severely disfiguring the woman. Despite the praise and protestations by high-profile women like Carol Doda, the San Francisco exotic dancer known for her enormous breasts, the systemic reactions to silicone oil were so dangerous and alarming that during the early 1960s the Nevada legislature made silicone breast injections a felony. California followed suit, making injections a misdemeanor offense (Simon, 1995: 141).

Long before any breast implant litigation and FDA regulation, scientists were investigating the safety of silicone. During the 1940s, Dow Chemical scientists conducted the first significant research on the health effects of exposure to commercial silicone. These findings were first published in 1948 in an article entitled "Toxicological Studies on Certain Commercial Silicones and Hydrolyzable Silane Intermediates" in which commercial (as opposed to industrial) silicones were described as "physiologically inert" and "present no hazards" (Plaintiffs' Trial Statement, 1995:2). Unfortunately, this erroneous conclusion came to be cited and relied on by the manufacturers as well as the medical community. Another article published in 1950, "Toxicological Studies on Certain Commercial Silicones," reported that the silicone product being studied demonstrated no adverse health effects in rats who were fed the silicone (Mahlum Memorandum, Factual Cite, 1995:12). This 1948 article was known as the seminal article on the potential health hazards of silicone for the following forty years, being cited more than one hundred times (Plaintiffs' Trial Statement, 1995:13).

In the early 1950s, scientists for Dow Chemical were aware of potential human toxicity from silicone-related products. Silica was found to have "quite a high order of toxicity from dust inhalation," including such effects as breathing problems, central nervous system problems, depression and neuromuscular coordination problems" (Mahlum Memorandum, Factual Cite, 1995:15). In another study conducted in 1955, one of Dow Chemical's leading scientists, V. K. Rowe, concluded that silica was "capable of causing diffuse cellular infiltration and fibrotic changes in the lungs and other organs of certain types of animals" (Mahlum Memorandum, Factual Cite, 1995:19). During the 1950s and 1960s as well, Dow Chemical conducted hundreds of tests on silicones, many of which were reported in internal documents only and never published. Dow reached the conclusion that silicone was not inert and was biologically active in the human body, and caused adverse health effects such as decreased testicular size and reduced spermatogenesis (Plaintiffs' Trial Statement, 1995:19).

In one of its highly confidential reviews of its internal studies of silicone, termed the "Medtox Project," Dow Corning's principal conclusion was that there were sufficient deficiencies in the studies to limit the value of relying on their initial studies on the systemic effects of silicone in the body (Plaintiffs' submission to the National Science Panel, 1997).

In 1956, Dow Chemical discovered that liquid silicone traveled to the intestines, adrenal glands, skin, heart, skull, bones, brain, kidney, and other organs of rats. In lactating dogs, it traveled to the skin and hair, liver, kidney, pancreas, thyroid, spleen, and other organs, as well as the breast milk and urine. Dow Chemical never disclosed the true ramifications of this important research, which indicated that the fluid comprising 80 percent of the gel in implants migrated to the major organs of the body (Plaintiffs' Trial Statement, 1995:20). Although this knowledge was available, no one was informed of these effects. The silence of Dow Corning and Dow Chemical allowed the myth that silicone was inert to continue unchallenged. In 1959, Dow Chemical's Annual Report hid the reality of which they were aware, reporting that "because of their chemical inertness and lack of toxicity, silicones are rapidly finding use in medical research."

As early as 1961, Dow Corning researchers advised doctors developing implants that silicone leaked through the shell. Dow, concerned about this finding because of what it knew about the lethal results of silicone injections, concluded that this free silicone would have a very similar effect. One internal memo written by a Dow Corning marketing executive, Charles Leach, warned that

> Several of our customers, looking to us as leaders in the industry, asked me what we were doing. I assured them, with crossed fingers, that Dow Corning too had an active "contracture/gel migration" study underway. This apparently satisfied them for the moment, but one of these days they will be asking us for the results of our studies. (Byrne, 1996b:79)

Throughout the early 1960s, there was extensive national coverage of the adverse reactions of silicone injections, which included silicone fluid made by Dow Corning. Dow Corning learned from published newspaper and magazine articles as well as legislative hearings that silicone fluids were being injected for breast augmentation and that death and serious injury could result (Mahlum Memorandum, 1995:20). Articles in such popular magazines as *Harper's Bazaar* (October 19, 1964) and *Vogue* (September 28, 1964) reported in the early sixties that injected silicone fluids could migrate, harden, enter the bloodstream, and cause embolisms. Dow Corning is in fact quoted in the *Harper's Bazaar* article as saying that "only specifically tested and specially controlled (Dow Corning silicone fluid)—should be employed for injection purposes." In response to the very damaging press it was getting about the "disastrous results" and "horrors of injection," Dow Corning formed a "Silicone Injection Committee" consisting of nationally known and prominent medical doctors who met in Midland, Michigan, home of both Dow Corning and Dow Chemical Company, to look into the problem.

In the late 1960s, Dow Corning experienced not only bad press but also criminal indictments for illegally delivering into interstate commerce an unapproved drug—"Dow Corning Medical Fluid No. 360." An article in *The Washington Post* on August 17, 1967 reported that the drug was being used to enlarge women's breasts. This was not the first time Dow Corning had received negative press for using an unapproved drug to augment women's breasts and other parts of their bodies. During the latter part of 1963 and early 1964, physicians were injecting the silicone fluid into human beings in the course of removing facial wrinkles and contouring other parts of the body, besides augmenting women's breasts (Plaintiffs' Trial Statement, 1995:49–50). The FDA made it clear in 1965 that it, "regarded silicone fluid for injection as a new drug since it is not generally recognized among experts, qualified by scientific training and experience to evaluate its safety and effectiveness, as safe and effective for injection purposes" (Saduak, 1965). Because drugs such as silicone were regulated by the FDA in the 1960s while medical devices were not, Dow Corning and Drs. Cronin and Gerow developed an implant to hold the fluid. This thin, fragile silicone elastomer, "similar to plastic wrap" held the silicone fluid which was then inserted directly into the mammary area, a procedure that had been forbidden for silicone injections. (Plaintiffs' submission and proposed findings, 1997).

Dow Chemical and Dow Corning knew as early as 1965 that low molecular weight compounds in the silicone fluid in breast implants could pass through the breast implant shell and into the body, and they knew these compounds could be "absorbed, metabolized and were biologically mobile within the body" (Mahlum Memorandum, 1995:55–56). Dow Corning's own animal studies with free silicone gel indicated that free gel was too dangerous and was damaging to humans (Jenny, 1994), causing concern about potential migration. 3M/McGhan too knew of serious failures of its products and the risks of free silicone in tissue, but it concealed this information. Don McGhan wrote to Dr. Michael Purdue on May 20, 1976. "Your desire to have a soft mammary implant is getting a bit out of hand . . . the tissue strength of the bag has been reduced" (MDL-926 Silicone Breast Implant Litigation, MCG 14431–14432).

Despite possible problems associated with silicone, Dow Corning was convinced that there could be a world market for a procedure to enlarge women's breasts, using a product, silicone, that mimicked the natural feel of breast tissue. The Dow Corning Center for Aid to Medical Research, headed by Silas Braley, worked with Dr. Thomas Cronin, a professor at Baylor University and his resident, Dr. Frank Gerow, who were initially interested in developing a bag, similar to that which held blood, to hold a saline solution, thereby overcoming the problems associated with injected silicone. Dr. Braley had been approached by other researchers with suggestions for developing breast implants but was less than enthusiastic about their designs. For example, the suggestion of using sponges in the breast was deemed unacceptable because the breast tissue would grow into and merge with the sponge. Although this risk was unacceptable, Bristol-Myers Squibb would later develop a polyurethane foam-covered breast implant specifically designed so that the breast tissue would grow into it and merge with it. Many of these cases will be tried during the first half of 1998.

Braley worked with Gerow and Cronin, encouraging them to develop a silicone implant that would duplicate the feel of the normal breast, that would not deteriorate, and that would not travel through the body as silicone injections were known to do. Based on Dow Chemical's short-term tests and recommendations on the safety of silicone fluids from 1940 to 1962, the first silicone gel implant manufactured by Dow Corning was implanted in the human body in 1962, even though there had been no animal tests. Silas Braley indicated that no animal tests were necessary because the silicone itself had already been extensively tested. Dow Corning, having no chemical testing facilities of its own, entered into "secrecy agreements" with Dow Chemical on joint research and commercial development of silicone gel breast implants.

The Cronin implant, developed in 1962, consisted of about 55 percent silicone (between a quarter and a third of a quart of liquid silicone in gel form), along with other chemicals and liquids contained in a silastic membrane or elastomer composed mainly of silicone or silica (Bonavoglia, 1996b). A patch of Dacron was cemented to the back of these older implants to improve adhesion to the chest wall. These early implants were harder and more durable than the implants to come and looked like slightly flattened cylinders. After the first implant surgeries in 1962, both Cronin and Gerow worked with Braley to convince Dow Corning to make the implants available as medical devices. Other companies soon began to market implants, including the Natural Y, Même, Replicon, Vogue, and Optimum. Surgitek Company, presently a subsidiary of Bristol-Myers Squibb, began manufacturing a particular type of implant with a polyurethane plastic foam coating, preferred by some surgeons because the foam meshed with human tissue, seemingly reducing the problem of capsular contracture—fairly common for women with gel implants. Unfortunately the polyurethane implants, implanted in approximately three hundred thousand women, some of whom had mastectomies because of a cancer risk, were found to contain the chemical 2–4 toluenediamine (TDA), a known animal carcinogen, and were removed from the market even before the FDA restrictions on implants.

Capsular contractures, which cause unnatural hardness and tightness of the breast, were and remain a serious and painful local complication of implants. Some researchers describe contractures, when the implant becomes surrounded by scar tissue inside the body, as the body's "natural" response to a foreign body. Others see it as resulting from bleeding, infection, or silicone leakage. One contracture is often followed by another, necessitating numerous and frequently ineffective surgeries in which the tissue capsule is removed or the entire implant is replaced (U.S. Congress, 1993:6). Some plastic surgeons avoid surgery by using "closed capsulotomy," which as noted earlier is the technique of placing a woman's contracted breast between the palms of their hands and force-fully squeezing and pressing from the outside until the capsule breaks (and the woman's breasts are black and blue), informally referred to as the "nutcracker technique."

Dow Corning had been aware of many of the risks and problems as-sociated with breast implants since 1948 (and other manufacturers since 1956). Despite this, silicone gel implants entered the market and re-mained on the market totally untested, unregulated, and unproven. Dr. Cronin, who had developed the first silicone implant, presented a paper on the development of silicone gel breast implants to the American So-ciety of Plastic and Reconstructive Surgeons in 1963 indicating his *belief* that they were safe. His status as a professor and a respected surgeon provided credibility to his claim, evidently calming any doubts others might have. Dow Corning thereafter operated under the formal but false assumption that silicone was a biologically inert substance. Hence, even if there were to be leakage from the implant, the fluid that escaped and migrated to distant sites would do no harm to the body's tissues. It is difficult to understand how such a contention could be taken seriously when liquid silicone had been banned and its use made a felony. Dow Corning was aware of a 1952 article published in the *Stanford Medical Bulletin* reporting "widespread" toxic manifestations in rabbits fed a high cholesterol diet containing DC 200 silicone fluid, including renal damage and kidney lesions (Cutting, 1952).

Salespeople and surgeons became increasingly concerned about the inescapable fact that silicone implants seeped or bled. The implants tended to develop an oily film, a tacky substance on their surface after being manipulated. Responding to potential sales problems (not, how-ever, to potential dangers to the women who would have these in their bodies), Tom Salisbury, a marketing representative for Dow Corning, recommended that sales staff visit the restroom and wash the implants with soap and water immediately before showing them to plastic sur-geons (Angell, 1996). One physician, Henry Jenny, was so concerned about the "bleed" or leaking of silicone from the implant that he devel-oped a saline implant as early as 1967 and worked with the Heyer-Schulte Corporation to have it on the market by 1968. Heyer-Schulte manufactured these implants, and Dr. Jenny bought the first two hun-dred for use in his own practice. Had saline implants been heavily pro-moted and marketed like silicone implants later were, the implant crisis might not be so severe. While the outer shell of saline implants is made of silicone and can cause problems in susceptible women, the degree and severity of problems associated with saline implants is much less than silicone implants, in which both the shell and the entire contents are silicone, although there remains serious concern about the consequences of ruptured saline implants.

THE MIDDLE YEARS: COMPETITION AND GROWING CONCERNS

Throughout the 1970s and 1980s, thousands of women each month were being supplied with one of several varieties of implants that the manufacturers marketed heavily and promoted to plastic surgeons through medical journals as well as sales representatives. Because implants were touted as perfectly safe, physicians and women expressed no reluctance about using them for augmentation as well as for reconstruction after mastectomy (U.S. Congress, 1993). While making safety claims, manufacturers harbored some concerns. An internal 3M memo in 1977 declared that "virtually no documented safety and efficacy data exist on (McGhan's) implant products—I'm only pointing out that serious deficiencies appear to exist with his products from the documentation standpoint" (U.S. Congress, 1993).

From 1963 until the very recent past, implants were marketed as a lifetime product, but there was no parallel lifetime testing. While Dow Corning's representatives insisted that they "thought" implants were safe, they admitted, as Silas Braley said, that "there were no tests for implant materials either on the material or on the patient, on the animal. All we could do was put it in and look and see what happens. There were no standards. There were no protocols. There was nothing" (Byrne, 1996a).

The best 3M could do was report as they did in the Harris County, Texas trials, that they had "no knowledge" of the potential health hazard (gel rupture, bleed, and migration) posed to women. The Même implant too was inadequately studied, relying on an eighteen month follow-up of 81 Même recipients in one case and short cut animal studies in another. But even more disturbing is the fact that the polyurethane foam used in the implants was created for furniture upholstery, oil filters, and carburetors, and its medical use was completely unmonitored for eight years. Ed Griffiths, a product manager at Scotfoam Corporation, the foam's manufacturer, was shocked to discover that its foam was not being used for an industrial application. "My eyes popped out when Powell (a Cooper Surgical vice president) explained his company was buying the foam from a jobber in Los Angeles and using it as a covering for a breast implant. They had been using our foam for many years, and it was the first time that I or anyone else at the company had heard about it" (Regush 1992:29).

The few brands of implants that were tested before marketing and distribution were only tested in animals in very limited and methodologically flawed studies. Still, the results of these limited tests were alarming, showing disease, silicone migration, and frequent deaths in the animals that were implanted and studied.

A review of the research on breast implants between 1970 and 1990 reveals a pattern in which one technique or type of implant was lauded, often by its developer, as a new and improved version, only to be condemned later and replaced by the "new and improved product," (Simon, 1995) a pattern repeated numerous times. To make implants that both looked and felt like real breasts, a number of different implant combinations were created: the "double lumen" implant that is much like one implant inside another, a triple lumen gel-filled implant surrounded by a saline outer layer, and others. At one point, implants with Dacron patches on the back to adhere to the woman's chest wall were applauded until it was discovered that the Dacron disintegrated in the patient's body. The Même implant was developed in 1982 by Bristol-Myers Squibb to overcome the hardening and breaking problems of other implants. It consisted of a silicone-gel sac with a polyurethane foam cover. The Même quickly captured a large share of the implant market, in part due to the sophisticated advertising and marketing of its developer, Harold Markham, and partly because of its similarity to the Natural-Y, a foam covered implant developed for mastectomy patients. Plastic surgeons relied on the company's promotional literature and simply assumed it was safe. As one plastic surgeon stated, "Because the Même was supposedly an improved design, we assumed it was probably safe. All we really knew is what the company told us" (Regush, 1992:28). Polyurethane foam-covered implants were acclaimed until it was discovered later, after tens of thousands of women had them, that the polyurethane disintegrated into the carcinogen TDA in the body, and that the polyurethane adhered to the woman's body in such a way that it could not be removed without disfiguring surgery (U.S. Congress, 1993:11). The number of manufacturers involved in the production of implants, each claiming superiority to the next, continued to increase, so that by 1990 there were seven major implant manufacturers making about forty types of implants, almost all silicone gel filled. The *Annals of Plastic Surgery* and *Plastic & Reconstructive Surgery* throughout the seventies and eighties carried full-page advertisements touting the advantages of one implant over another.

Rather than test implants for safety, the process of introducing chemicals (silicone, silica, liquid silicone, and polyurethane) into women's bodies was one of cooperative give and take between plastic surgeons and the manufacturers, one in which women served as a testing ground. Manufacturers worked with plastic surgeons to perfect the implants, taking suggestions from surgeons about the problems their patients were experiencing back to the drawing board, refining or redesigning the implants, and again providing them for doctors. This process continued well into the late 1980s. Dr. Richard Grossman, a plastic surgeon and author of an early text on how to perform breast augmentation surgery, notified the FDA in 1989 that "For years it has been the custom and practice of manufacturers to modify the implants based on ideas of surgeons, and then provide these custom-made prototypes that would be tried out on patients to see how they worked" (U.S. Congress, 1993:13). No animal studies of these modified prototypes were conducted before implanting them into women. Dr. Grossman admitted to the FDA that he had participated in four such "studies" but had stopped because they seemed unethical and because the complication rate (20 to 25 percent) was unacceptably high (U.S. Congress, 1993:13).

Along with maintaining this hand-in-glove relationship with manufacturers, plastic surgeons continued to present a far rosier picture of the safety and longevity of implants than any of the clinical or research findings warranted. During the mid-1970s, Dow Corning knew that some doctors were cutting implants open and inserting the silicone gel directly into the woman's body. They then studied the possibility of an implantable silicone gel but concluded it was impossible. The gel migrated and there were significant problems with microparticularization, in which the silicone continues to break down into smaller and smaller parts, leading to chronic inflammation.

Dow Corning had 100 percent of the breast implant market until the early 1970s, when McGhan Medical (purchased in 1977 by 3M Corporation) and Heyer-Schulte Corporation (now owned by Baxter Corporation) became worrisome competitors. These corporations advertised heavily for a larger share of the market; in one issue of *Plastic and Reconstructive Surgery* (March 1976), while Dow Corning celebrated the wide choice available to surgeons and women (a total of twenty-six sizes in four designs, including low-profile round, round, low-profile contour, contour), Heyer-Schulte stressed the strength and durability of its implants as well as the convenience of custom design, through their "People Helping People personal service" ads. At the same time however, they acknowledged "problems associated with physical migration including liver dysfunction and foreign body granuloma in four victims of silicone injection . . . [and] similar mononuclear and giant cell reaction results in some patients wherein silicone gel has escaped from the shell" (MDL-926 Silicone Breast Implant Litigation, Baxter 83650–83652).

As Heyer-Schulte and McGhan began to compete successfully for a larger share of the growing implant market, Dow responded by developing an implant with a much thinner shell and more fluid gel in hopes of regaining the market it was losing. The new implants were designed to overcome an appearance problem. While they looked lifelike when a woman was sitting or standing, when she lay down they spread across her chest too much, flattening her appearance. As Corning's James Baker opined, when the woman was supine, she looked like "Mount Vesuvius" (Byrne, 1996a:49). To create a more lifelike implant, both the envelope that contained the gel and the gel itself were made thinner, now containing about 75 percent gel instead of 55 percent, which earlier implants had. While this change may have enhanced the appearance and created a more natural looking implant, the result was a greater possibility of leakage or rupture, allowing greater opportunity for the liquid silicone in silicone gel to travel throughout the body.

In 1975, in fact, Dow Corning chemical engineers who were working on Dow Corning research specialist Arthur Rathjen's task force to create a new generation of more competitive, lighter implants, expressed their concern "about a possible bleed situation" with the new gel but continued to promote implants as safe and gel as inert, based on an imperfect and outdated 1948 study (Rowe et al.), even though they were aware that the FDA had banned the use of liquid silicone in the human body in the early 1960s (U.S. Congress, 1993). Henry Jenny was concerned enough about problems with the implants to speak to the FDA advisory panel at their meeting in Washington in 1978 about the similarities between silicone injected in the body and silicone lost from an intact implant by gel bleed. He was not talking about problems associated with rupture, but about the *normal, predictable, and anticipated* seepage of gel from the intact implant, a seepage that made the implant moist and sticky.

3M/McGhan also knew that gel bleed of silicone posed dangers. A June 9, 1981 technical report summary by R.L. Knoll entitled "Trimester Technical Report" on silicone gel diffusion stated: "Histological studies suggest that gel bleed of silicone has been found in the capsule and may be a 'prime candidate' causing or contributing to capsular contracture" (MDL-926 Silicone Breast Implant Litigation, MMM 4960–4962). Acknowledging that it should develop a method to quantitatively determine the amount of gel bleed, 3M/McGhan finally concluded such testing was simply "not worth the effort" (Plaintiffs' Response to Defendants, 1996:4).

Dow Corning was aware of criticisms directed against it but was undeterred from pursuing the manufacture of a silicone gel implant. In 1977, Arthur Rathjen wrote that Dow Corning had experienced "strict criticism by the American Society of Plastic and Reconstructive Surgeons (ASPRS) because of our position with the silicone fluid injection program." Rathjen further noted: "When we first got involved with the A.S.P.R.S. with the silicone symposium, we were accused as a corporation of disregarding safety and efficacy data to jam our product through so that we could recoup [sic] some of our investment dollars and we were looked at as a large corporation who disregarded safety and efficacy standards to make money" (Mahlum Memorandum, Factual Cite, 1995:48–49). He was clearly concerned about the lack of knowledge Dow Corning still had about bleed. In 1976 he wrote: "We better get going on a basic long-range project relative to gel, its formulation, toxicology, etc., over and above what is now underway." He further worried: "Is there something in the implant that migrates out or off the mammary prosthesis? Yes or no! Does it continue for the life of the implant, or is it limited or controlled for a period of time? Does it come from the envelope, or gel, or both?" Rathjen concluded with the question that revealed the unbelievable lack of knowledge held by a manufacturer producing a medical device to be placed in the human body: "What is it?" (Angell, 1996:60). Rathjen's concerns at Dow Corning were matched with the fears of some plastic surgeons. In a September 27, 1976 letter to Don McGhan, President of McGhan Medical Corporation, Dr. A. Michael Pardue outlined the severe problems his patients experienced. For example, when removing a silicone gel breast implant he found it was ruptured, with "just a large gelatinous mass in which it was difficult to distinguish the implant cover. The tag had pulled away from the implant, the lining of the tissue capsule was inflated and was a purplish-red color." He concludes, "Don, this case today was one of the most frightening cases I have ever had. The inflammatory and scar tissue response to the ruptured implant was incredible. Therefore, I am returning all McGhan implants which we have not used to you for a full refund" (Pardue, 1976).

A 1978 study undertaken by Medical Engineering Corporation, a company later sold to Bristol-Myers Squibb, revealed that such adverse reactions as "hemorrhage, possible pneumonia, and hyperplasia of the lymphoid tissue in the large intestine" appeared in implanted dogs. In their effort to deny safety problems and destroy evidence of the danger of silicone, before FDA inspectors arrived at the plant, the company president responded with a memo commanding "Destroy dogs ASAP" and later, "kill dogs, forget organs, just dispose of them" (U.S. Congress, 1993:35). These dogs were sick, and their organs were filled with silicone that had migrated from their implants.

It wasn't just that some scientists were expressing significant concern about the possible negative consequences of silicone gel, or that they knew it migrated to the liver and other organs. In the late 1960s and early 1970s, scientists knew that certain silicone compounds possessed sufficient biological activity to have potential use as pharmaceuticals. Dow Corning, as early as 1970, had found inflammatory reactions in dog studies, and some Dow scientists were concerned about the possibility of breakage or leakage of breast implants. Dow Chemical, far from believing that silicone was inert, was involved in research designed to develop it as a drug and an insecticide. Studies done on silicone compounds described it as "endowed with a potential depressant activity on [the] central nervous system" (Mahlum Memorandum, 1995:53). This knowledge that silicones used in medical products were not inert was largely concealed and withheld from the public and the medical community by Dow Corning and Dow Chemical for more than twenty-five years.

THE FDA: HESITATION AND INACTION

Manufacturers were becoming increasingly aware of the FDA's growing concern about the lack of safety testing and faced the great likelihood that implants would soon be regulated. Following the furor over the Dalkon Shield intrauterine device, in 1976 the FDA had received authority to regulate medical devices under the Medical Device Amendments to the Food, Drug and Cosmetics Act (Public Law 94–295, in Simon, 1995:148). Implant manufacturers raced against the inevitable requirement of safety testing to get their implants on the market. Chemical engineer Tom Talcott, for example, wrote in 1975 that the Dow Corning Mammary Task Force, of which he was a member—"moved to accelerate the new fluid gel filled breast implant introduction and was successful in beating device regulation to obtain 'grandfather' status" (Chestney, 1994:3).

As it turned out, the legislation introduced in 1976 had a very limited impact on safety testing because it did not apply to implants that were on the market through 1976, and it exempted all post–1976 implants that were not substantially different from those already in existence. Therefore, only a fraction of the implants on the market were required to undergo the regulatory practice of premarket approval; all others were effectively grandfathered in without regulation.

Throughout the seventies and into the early eighties, even as manufacturers rushed to get implants on the market, questions about the safety of silicone generally and implants specifically continued to surface, now with increasing frequency. Not surprisingly, the efforts of manufacturers to avoid regulation and to convince the plastic surgeons of the safety of implants increased as well. In April 1982, manufacturers met for two days to brainstorm ways to convince the FDA to delay regulating implants. They were aware of the significant problems. In 1980 for example, in a letter to its sales representatives, a Surgitek spokesperson wrote, "Regrettably one of the characteristics of silicone rubber is that it has a very low tear strength. Even if Dow Corning has made a shell with twice the tear strength of what they presently have the new value will still be low compared to other materials such as Saran Wrap" (Lynch and Stith *Surgitek* memo to field force, MDL-926 Silicone Breast Implant Litigation depository 7056).

Growing concerns about breast implants led the FDA panel to consider classifying breast implants as a Class III medical device along with silicone injections, which had immediately been classified as Class III with the passage of the 1976 Medical Device Amendments Law (Public Law 94–295). However, the panel, which included a number of plastic surgeons, recommended a Class II classification, one requiring less stringent safety testing. Finally, the FDA, evidently convinced by manufacturers and plastic surgeons that implants had been used safely for ten years, did not classify them, allowing them to remain on the market virtually unregulated, with no requirement for any safety or efficacy testing.

With mounting concern from consumers and some physicians about silicone gel-filled implants, the FDA Plastic Surgery Device Panel held a meeting in 1983 about silicone breast implants and issued a final recommendation to classify silicone gel breast implants as Class III devices. This classification required the most stringent regulation and the most careful proof of safety, indicating that the FDA assumed implants had a potential for unreasonable risk of injury to humans. Dr. Norman Anderson, who chaired the panel from 1981 to 1983, said about the decision:

At that time there were great worries about the sufficiency of data to establish the safety and efficacy of this product. The manufacturers and the American Society of Plastic and Reconstructive Surgeons, and the FDA made a commitment in the public register and to the public to resolve, at that time, the void in data. (Chestney, 1994:38)

Anderson again chaired the Plastic Surgery Device Panel in 1988 and reported:

At that time, the issues were somewhat different than in 1982; but again the same coalition came forward (ASPRS and manufacturers). There was an agreement on the floor that the plastic surgery society would work with the FDA to establish a registry, and we would find new information to deal with the tremendous void in sufficiency of data. This coalition disbanded when the Advisory Panel left the room. (Chestney, 1994:38)

So, despite the concern about fibrous capsular contractures, silicone leakage, migration of silicone from bleed and rupture, infection, interference with breast tumor detection, carcinogeneity, autoimmune disease, and calcification, the "tremendous void" in safety information was still not addressed in any systematic fashion until after 1988. However, even after all the delay in requiring safety testing, the manufacturers were allowed nearly three more years to provide valid scientific evidence showing that there was a reasonable assurance of the safety of breast implants.

By June 1988, when the FDA finally determined that it did not have enough information to assure the safety of breast implants, they had been on the market for almost twenty-five years, long enough for many women to exhibit serious problems. And indeed the FDA had heard from thousands of women about problems with implants. These problems included fatigue, headaches, nausea, flu-like symptoms, scleroderma, esophageal immotility, dry mucous membranes, hair loss, memory loss, and other problems. Women were presenting these problems to their doctors and were often misdiagnosed or diagnosed as suffering from emotional problems because of the number and range of symptoms they presented. Physicians were not aware of a syndrome that reflected the vast number of symptoms these women had and were faced with a plethora of symptoms that looked very much like other diseases, but did not meet all of the criteria for being classified as any of them, such as rheumatism, arthritis, lupus, and defined neurological disorders.

Dow Corning, meanwhile, was aware from its own research that there were problems with the implants. Thus, even though there was no requirement yet to prove the safety of implants in order to keep them on the market, the company took action to protect itself. In 1985 Dow Corning, still the largest manufacturer of silicone implants, rewrote the product warnings that accompanied the packaged implants to warn of possible autoimmune risks with silicone gel implants. These inserts were provided to the surgeon and were Dow Corning's effort to transfer the responsibility for implants from the manufacturer to the physician. This 1985 change supplemented the mild warnings already provided with the implants, indicating that localized reactions, capsular contractures or hardening of the breast tissue, and loss of nipple sensitivity were possible side effects.

In addition to the insert, Dow later advertised in the *Journal of Plastic and Reconstructive Surgery* (1988) that its implants came with a warranty: "Dow Corning now offers a limited warranty on SILASTIC brand mammary implants. This implant warranty program which we are calling P.R.E.P. for Product Replacement Expense Program will provide assistance to the uninsured patient should there be a loss of shell integrity within 5 years of implantation." This warranty provides not only "replacement implants" but also "up to $600.00 in Operating Room and/ or Surgeon's Fees."

In 1990, the American Society of Plastic and Reconstructive Surgeons published a brochure entitled "Straight Talk About Breast Implants," which included a good deal of misinformation about the longevity and safety of both saline and silicone implants, information that came directly, and without substantial verification, from manufacturers. The fact that breast implants often constituted a significant portion of the plastic surgeons' annual revenues likely encouraged them to accept the salespersons' assertions without any investigation on their own.

Not only did the manufacturers and the plastic surgeons make every effort to keep implants on the market and unregulated despite clear evidence of lack of safety data, but the FDA also kept secret hundreds of studies of gel implants that had been conducted by Dow Corning. In November 1990, U.S. District Judge Stanley Sporkin ordered the FDA to make public animal studies dating back to the 1960s that Dow Corning had delivered to the agency. Sporkin criticized the FDA's agreement with Dow Corning to protect the confidentiality of these documents as a ruse to avoid the Freedom of Information Act. Even the FDA's own scientific advisory panel was not given internal Dow Corning documents that addressed the real and potential dangers of breast implants and silicone. These documents, dating from 1962–1980, had been under court seal, even though their contents had been referred to at previous FDA meetings and subcommittee hearings. They indicated that Dow Corning had suspected for years that the implants were not as safe as they maintained in public (Ingersoll, 1992). It was not until February 1992, under intense pressure following extensive media coverage, that Dow Corning publicly released these documents, revealing the company's knowledge of bleed, inflammation, and migration for the first time (U.S. Congress, 1993). An

FDA consultant, who reviewed 10,000 pages of Dow Corning documents, insisted that the lack of relevant scientific studies was astonishing (Hilts, 1992).

In December 1990, Representative Ted Weiss, chair of the Human Resources and Intergovernmental Relations Subcommittee of the Committee on Government Operations, conducted a hearing on the FDA's regulation of breast implants. At these hearings, representatives of every interest group related to implants made their cases to the Committee. These included not only the usual players, the plastic surgeons and manufacturers, but now contingents of sick and disfigured women as well as women paid by the ASPRS to attend the meetings and tell of the need to keep implants on the market.

This investigation concluded that the FDA itself had been insensitive to the complaints of consumers. Riddled with internal politics, the FDA had bowed to the demands of the well-funded ASPRS and manufacture lobbyists. The agency, the investigation revealed, was sullied by conflicts of interest of the members participating on the medical devices panel, many of whom were plastic surgeons with ties to manufacturers.

Furthermore, the investigation concluded that the FDA had misled the public about the safety of implants for fifteen years, and had wrongly made public statements about breast implants which minimized the risks known to be associated with silicone implants. Even this investigation of the FDA and the conclusions that it had failed to protect the public did not result in adequate monitoring of the implants. The cover letter that accompanied the Committee on Government Operations' report of its investigation of the FDA states: "Unfortunately, our investigation indicates that the FDA *continues* (author's emphasis) to fail to safeguard implant patients, making it very important that this report be released in a timely manner" (U.S. Congress, 1993:v).

By the time David Kessler severely restricted the sale of silicone breast implants in April 1992, they had been on the market in the United States for almost three decades. During that time, over eight hundred thousand women had received implants. Hundreds of thousands of implants had also been sold overseas. In addition, many women had had more than one set of implants due to rupture, contracture, or other problems. The actual number of women with implants is unknown; manufacturers prefer to use the figure of 2 million in order to minimize the rate of problems, including contracture, rupture, and autoimmune responses; consumer groups and breast implant support groups assume the number to be somewhat less than 1 million. The actual number of implants manufactured and sold has never been documented, largely because the manufacturers refuse to create a registry of their products sold, which would allow the rate of problems with implants to be tracked.

During these decades, women were not aware that they were being used as test animals in implant research and knew nothing about any risks tied to the silicone being placed in their bodies. Almost without exception, the women we interviewed were told that their implants were "one hundred percent safe," "would not rupture unless they were hit by a truck," and "would last a lifetime." Doctors sometimes went to great lengths to convince their patients of the implants' safety, assuring them that "you will go to your graves with perky breasts," or throwing the implants against their office walls to demonstrate their strength and elasticity. These women had no reason to be concerned about the safety of implants. As Dow Corning, in a full-page ad in the *Annals of Plastic Surgery* (1983) featuring the implant it introduced in 1962, boasted: "By the way, our first implants are still in place today." It is probably not as surprising to most readers that Dow Corning and other manufacturers heavily marketed their implants to plastic surgeons as it is to realize that these physicians relied almost exclusively on the manufacturers' salespersons and advertising brochures in their evaluation of the implants. As noted earlier, physicians passed on to women the false information that these implants were safe while requiring absolutely no documentation of their safety. This inexcusable carelessness would prove devastating for many women.

The conclusion that manufacturers acted in a reprehensible manner toward the women of this country is inescapable. Congressman Ted Weiss's investigation draws several conclusions that illustrate this point. Because the findings of this investigation were so important, they are presented in summary form below (U.S. Congress, 1993).

1. The FDA ignored warnings about the need to regulate breast implants for over a decade. As early as 1978, scientists and physicians discussed their concerns about the safety of breast implants with the FDA advisory committee, and by 1980 they were aware of all the problems that led to their removal from the market in 1992. As late as the 1980s, Dow Corning continued to rely on research that had been conducted by Industrial Biotech Lab in 1975 to demonstrate the safety of silicone gel, despite the fact that the study had to be abandoned because the FDA itself cited it as highly flawed, if not outright fraudulent. The study was inadequate to provide "reasonable assurance of the safety and effectiveness" of breast implants. In addition, methodological flaws led to an underestimation of both the type and rate of complications. The FDA was also informed that manufacturers were hiding safety information

from the doctors, the public, and the FDA. Although the advisory panel recommended the establishment of a national registry of implant patients who could then be followed long term, as well as a mandatory program to inform the public of the risks, the manufacturers and plastic surgeons successfully defeated these recommendations.

2. Scientists have been concerned about the risks of connective tissue and autoimmune disorders related to breast implants since 1975. Surgitek and other companies were aware of possible "antibody reaction from an immunological response" as early as 1977, and in 1982 scientists at the University of Chicago reported that the body's reaction to silicone created giant cells called macrophages that erode the silicone envelope and cause silicone to migrate to the lymph nodes. Their request for funds from Dow Corning to study this process further was rejected. Based on a growing body of literature, FDA scientists reported that silicone could cause connective tissue disorders, also called autoimmune disorders, including potentially fatal diseases such as scleroderma. Dr. Nir Kossovsky, professor of pathology at UCLA, reported to the FDA in 1990 that silicone bleeds from intact implants. Dr. Frank Vasey, professor of medicine at the University of South Florida, reported that when his patients, suffering from such diseases as lupus, scleroderma, Sjögren's syndrome, arthritis and severe muscle pain, had their implants removed, 81 percent improved (U.S. Congress, 1993:16).

3. Physicians, engineers, and employees of implant manufacturers have been concerned about breakage and leakage of silicone gel implants, as well as the migration of gel to other organs, since the 1970s. In 1975, an internal memo from a Dow Corning task force mentioned the possible migration of gel found in one of its monkey tests. In 1979, Medical Engineering Corporation, later Surgitek, reported the results of a dog study that showed "low but definite concentrations of silicon in kidney and liver tissue" (U.S. Congress, 1993:19). Tom Talcott, a former Dow Corning engineer wrote, "We are hearing complaints from the field about the demonstration samples they are receiving. The general claim is that the units bleed profusely after they have been flexed vigorously." He then requested testing to determine if a bleed rate problem existed (17). In 1975, Arthur Rathjen wrote: "I have proposed again and again that we must begin an in depth study of our gel, envelope, and bleed phenomenon. Capsule contraction isn't the only problem. Time is going to run out on us if we don't get underway" (U.S. Congress, 1993:18). In December 1977, another internal Dow Corning memo, expressing concern about loss of business resulting from ruptures and "greasy implants," reported rupture problems encountered by four doctors ranging from 11 percent to 32 percent. Robinson et al. (1995) reported a 50 percent

rupture rate after only seven years of usage. Dr. Charles Vinnik wrote Dow Corning in 1981 about the "shell failure" of silicone implants and the reaction that was as profound as "anything we ever saw with the silicone injections." He described one implant as "totally disrupted with the implant shell incorporated within the gel mass" and a "roughly 4 × 6 cm irregular nodular mass," which was an "obvious siliconoma" (U.S. Congress, 1993:18).

In 1977, officials at Surgitek were concerned that silicone oil bleeding through the shell into the body tissue could cause the FDA to remove silicone gel implants from the market (U.S. Congress, 1993:19). Others questioned whether the hard squeezing exercises surgeons suggested to their patients to prevent capsular contracture would actually cause "progressive weakening and eventual rupture" of the implant (U.S. Congress, 1993:19), and one memo reported that any sort of rough handling would cause bleed. Despite their knowledge of the possible complications of silicone gel, its lack of inertness, and its medicinal and insecticide potential, the manufacturers continued to misinform and mislead the public and the FDA regarding rupture, contracture, and other complications. In 1992, the CEO of Dow Corning represented the failure rate of implants to be 0.5 percent (Jenny, 1994:151). Yet Dr. Frank Vasey, a respected physician and expert witness for the plaintiff, estimates that the current failure rate may be between 30 and 40 percent, and that eventually all implants will break or bleed (Vasey and Feldstein, 1993). Despite the degree of risk these manufacturers knew existed, as recently as 1991 anyone who called the Dow Corning Hot Line would be told that the research indicated that implants were 100 percent safe.

Dr. Pierre Blais, who investigated the safety of implants for the Canadian Department of National Health and Welfare, testified that the testing done on implants over the last decades was "trivial," if not totally irrelevant." He further stated that the implants' "performance is far below that of products used in other medical areas," that the shell and gel chemically change in the body, that the implants cannot sustain closed capsulotomies, and that the tissue around them forms an abrasive, sandpaper-like substance ensuring their deterioration and rupture. Dr. Donna de Camara, University of Illinois School of Medicine, reported data in 1991 showing that implants were likely to break as they aged, regardless of whether a woman experienced a trauma. In her study of thirty-one women (fifty-one implants), she found that twenty-seven (53 percent) were ruptured, an additional seven (14 percent) were leaking, and only seventeen (33 percent) were intact after seven or more years. Despite assurances that implants would last a lifetime, research reported by the American Society of Plastic and Reconstructive Surgery Educational Foundation shows that "implants made more than ten years ago and removed now are almost always broken."

4. The FDA ignored its own scientists' advice to reject manufacturers' premarket approval applications (PMAs) in 1991. The PMA applications were required of manufacturers to show that they had sufficient evidence of safety and efficacy for the FDA to conduct a review. If the FDA found the data to be insufficient, it could refuse to file the application, thereby preventing the manufacturer from selling the implants. The FDA scientists found the applications to be so methodologically flawed and grossly insufficient that they recommended that the FDA not file the applications. After manufacturers and plastic surgeons spent months lobbying the FDA and Congress, the scientists' recommendations were overruled by the FDA officials, with no written justifications for their actions. This was an unusual occurrence for any Health and Human Services agency.

5. Professional pro-implant lobbyists hired by manufacturers included former FDA officials and some former staff members of then President George Bush. The ASPRS hired three lobbying firms whose lobbyists included Mark Heller, formerly with the FDA, Deborah Steelman, former White House aide and then advisor to the president on health issues, Charles Black, former White House aide, and other well-connected people. In addition, the ASPRS paid for almost four hundred women to go to Washington and lobby their senators and representatives about the importance of breast implants. The ASPRS developed a model letter for their doctors, nurses, and patients to send to the FDA. The letter was based on incorrect and misleading information such as breast implants were being regulated more stringently than other medical devices and that media hysteria and a "few disgruntled patients" were behind the effort to remove implants from the market. Lobbyists also worked to remove members of the advisory committee who pressed for more regulation; they successfully removed Dr. Norman Anderson, former chair, as well as several others.

6. Manufacturers have never provided proof of the safety of implants to the FDA. Although companies knew at least since 1982 that they would be required to provide safety data, many of the studies were not started until 1990 and 1991. Several major problems plagued the studies that they finally conducted:

- Although implants are sold as a permanent medical device, most studied women for only two years or less, an absurdly insufficient time. There were no lifetime studies.

- In many of the studies, the majority of the women were not followed up after the first few months, so there was inadequate information to assess safety.

- In several studies, women were not asked about connective tissue/autoimmune disorders, cancer, or other medical problems associated with silicone breast implants. Often the research included only medical records of the plastic surgeons. Since women would not be likely to return to their plastic surgeon but rather to their general practitioner for other than directly related problems, the incidence of other common problems is underreported.

- The number of reconstruction patients in most studies was so small that they could not provide persuasive evidence of safety.

- Several companies did not study women with certain models of implants, simply generalizing from one model to others. Surprisingly, no studies were done on the degree of force required to rupture an implant.

- In addition to the problems with clinical studies, the animal studies presented numerous problems, including lack of followup, inadequate time, and the fact that implants were never placed beneath the breast tissue, tissue that is more sensitive than other kinds of tissue.

7. FDA officials and manufacturers prevented the 1991 breast implant advisory panel from considering crucial safety information. The panel determined that four manufacturers did not provide adequate safety and effectiveness information. Even so, they allowed them to continue to market the implants as a "public health necessity" because of lack of evidence of substantiated risks. Personal accounts of women from Y-Me took the place of such studies as that done by Dr. Donna de Camara, which concluded that implants were likely to break after seven years. The panel was not given this information, nor were the documents from Dow Corning which were kept sealed under court order made available. These documents, finally released after great public pressure, showed that Dow Corning scientists were well aware of and concerned about the lack of safety data and that they knew that the thinner implants were more inclined to break. Dow Corning was far more concerned about the impact of bleeding and breaking on sales than about the women's health. They failed to disclose study results showing inflammation of the lymph nodes and other symptoms that could indicate immune disorders. They reported few, if any, real problems to the FDA, and they excluded from their reports to the FDA any studies that showed problems. Furthermore, even though they were aware of problems in the animal studies, they

arranged to have implants put in women before the animal studies were completed, in violation of ethical standards for research on humans. It is shocking that the implants were kept on the market not because the panel thought they were safe, but because there were insufficient data to prove they were unsafe as a direct and premeditated result of corporate misconduct.

8. In 1991, FDA concerns about cancer led to the withdrawal of breast implants covered with polyurethane foam. These implants became popular in the late 1980s when they were produced by Cooper Surgical, which later sold its implant business to Surgitek. FDA investigators found that these implants were made under nonsterile conditions. For example, company employees blew into polyurethane foam implants to test for inflation (U.S. Congress, 1993:31). In 1990, an FDA scientist made the first public statement revealing that polyurethane used on the implants breaks down to form the carcinogenic TDA. By March 1991, an FDA scientist had warned that Surgitek had terminated a study that may have indicated a cancer risk from polyurethane foam. In May 1991, a scientist from Aegis Analytic Laboratory warned the FDA that it had conducted a study for Surgitek in which it had found TDA in the breast milk of implanted women. The scientist was concerned that the company was not making the information available to the public or to the FDA. Surgitek withdrew its polyurethane foam-covered implants from the market in 1991, but between 200,000 and 400,000 women had already received these implants between 1985 and 1990. Polyurethane foam-coated implants place the woman in double jeopardy: the foam meshes with human tissue and when these implants rupture, the foam has "disappeared"; yet the disfigurement to the chest is immense. It generally takes a surgeon an hour or two to remove a ruptured silicone implant from a woman, but if the implants are foam covered, the operation can take eight to ten hours.

9. The 1992 FDA advisory panel lacked crucial information about how breast implants interfere with mammography, a surgeon's ability to detect breast cancer, and other problems. Information that had been made available to the FDA about the impact of implants on mammograms was based more on opinion than on fact. Although there was very little published research on this matter, the FDA panel heard unsupported reports of new mammography techniques that were accurate for women with implants. One more accurate study indicated a significant reduction in the breast tissue which could be visualized with mammography, reducing the diagnostician's ability to detect breast cancer by 30 to 50 percent.

10. In 1992, Dow Corning disclosed that the company sold implants to doctors before they were shown to be safe even in animals, let alone

humans. Dow Corning submitted fabricated information about quality control. The FDA in 1992 expressed concern about the company's failure to report, as required under the Medical Devices Reporting (MDR) guidelines—problems such as capsular contractures, gel bleed, and other localized and systemic problems. There was deliberate and systematic underreporting of adverse reactions, as well as altering or replacing records to hide problems.

11. Patients have been misled about the safety of implants for at least the last fifteen years. Although breast implants were a common surgical procedure by the 1980s, Dow Corning knew in the 1970s that the FDA's imposition of a requirement for long term animal testing would cause the company problems. Internally characterizing this possibility as "ominous" for its interests, Dow Corning recognized that the silicone gel would not stand up to scrutiny; most of the safety claims were based on two-year dog studies that would not be approved under the lifetime test criterion, seven years for a dog study. Evidently, plastic surgeons relied completely on the salespersons and the company's brochures, which were in fact misleading or erroneous, including such statements as "loose silicone does not appear to be a health risk" and capsular contractures occur in about "one in ten women" (whereas research indicates at least a 30 to 40 percent contracture rate). Furthermore, Dow claimed that its "accurate information" about the safety of implants was based on "30 years of valid scientific research," a completely insupportable claim.

Through 1993, the plastic surgeons and manufacturers successfully fought the FDA's recommendation that all patients must receive all relevant safety information and warnings prior to surgery. Dow established a hot line that it advertised in newspapers all over the country so that women could call for "accurate" information. In fact, the information was inaccurate and dangerous, including: "scientific data and research show that they are 100 percent safe"; "We have done lengthy studies as have thousands of plastic surgeons to show that they are safe" (37); "there is no detrimental effect to having silicone in the body"; and "there has been significant testing on arthritis, scleroderma, lupus, and other problems with the immune system," showing that implants do not cause any immune system diseases or problems (37).

12. Even today, patients are still being misled by the FDA's approved informed consent form. The FDA's two-year attempt to have a cooperatively produced brochure on the safety and risks of implants failed, and it needed to develop an informed consent form to be used after 1992 for those patients who were having reconstruction. Medical associations and manufacturers continued to pressure the FDA to minimize the dangers in these forms and were able to force significant changes in wording and

...ning, partly by insisting that there "was no evidence" in situations in which they had refused to provide relevant evidence to the FDA through studies or documents. The FDA bowed to the manufacturers' will. Thus, the new warnings seriously underestimated the risks of which even the FDA was aware.

For example, the ASPRS requested the removal of statements such as: "Manufacturers have not provided the FDA adequate scientific evidence" of their safety and effectiveness, and "The number of women who now, or in the past, have had silicone gel-filled breast implants is not known. . . . It is also not known how many of these women have had problems" (38). These two statements were deleted and finally replaced with a far more positive statement: "Breast implants have been used in nearly two million women for nearly 30 years." The ASPRS also succeeded in replacing the statement that "closed capsulotomy must NOT be performed" with an advisory that it is not recommended. The FDA issued a strong warning about breast feeding on the informed consent form: "The surgical implantation of the device may interfere with a woman's ability to nurse her baby" (39). This warning was finally diluted to "Many women have nursed their babies successfully. . . . Any breast surgery could theoretically interfere with your ability to nurse your baby."

13. The FDA's public statements about breast implants minimized the risks associated with them. The agency continued to make public statements about the safety of breast implants, which were far more optimistic than its own scientists reported. Although the FDA's internal documents indicated insufficient evidence of safety to keep implants on the market, its public statements were more positive and supportive of manufacturers. For example, the FDA explained that Surgitek and Bristol-Myers Squibb, which manufactured the Même, had "voluntarily" removed polyurethane-covered implants from the market, when the FDA had strongly pressured them to do so. The FDA did not mention that the polyurethane foam was in fact Scott Industrial Foam, "a product made for automobile air filters and carpet cleaning equipment, never intended to be implanted in the human body" (41). Indeed, when Scott finally discovered that its industrial foam was being used to coat implants designed to be put inside the human body, the company's CEOs were appalled. It stopped selling this foam to Surgitek and instructed Surgitek to cease and desist using this foam as an implant cover. But Surgitek ignored Scott Foam's instructions and warnings and simply found another foam supplier.

14. FDA inspections in 1992 showed that the McGhan Corporation's production of breast implants had violated good manufacturing prac-

tices, but the FDA allowed McGhan to resume sales before the problem was corrected. In early 1992, only McGhan and Mentor (another breast implant manufacturer) were eligible to sell silicone gel breast implants, and an FDA investigation of McGhan found that the quality of the process used to verify confidence in the product was inadequate. The FDA concluded that in June of that year "conditions exist whereby there is a reasonable probability that unsafe or ineffective devices will be produced and distributed" (43). Although there is no evidence that McGhan implants are substantially different from or superior to Mentor implants, the FDA developed a "compassionate need exemption policy," evidently based on little other than a letter from one of the patients who was angry at having to wait so long for a McGhan implant. As a result, these implants remained on the market despite the problems in quality assurance.

15. From April 1992 to the present, the FDA has failed to adequately monitor the use of silicone breast implants, despite the promises of the FDA commissioner. The moratorium announced in 1992 contained an "urgent need" exemption to include women who needed their implants replaced because of rupture or contracture, mastectomy patients who were in the middle of a reconstruction process, and women who needed immediate reconstruction after mastectomy and were not candidates for saline implants. This was to be a temporary measure superseded by an "open availability research protocol" that could be developed for mastectomy patients and women with severe deformities. Although the FDA announced that it would require careful records on the women who received the implants and the surgeons who implanted them, as well as on the number of implants shipped by manufacturers, it never gathered such information and failed in its promise to "carefully monitor" their use. The FDA still does not require documentation from doctors which assures them that "deformity" is not defined so broadly as to include the pseudo-disease "hypomastia" (small breasts), which the ASPRS put forward in its efforts to legitimize increasing its profits.

This historical review documents the role of manufacturers and the FDA in this breast implant travesty. However, it is also necessary to look at the other side of this problem and to try to understand the cultural and social factors that make such damage to women possible in the first place. At the same time, just as when discussing rape or other forms of violence against women, we must not focus solely on women's decisions. These decisions must be placed in a context that acknowledges the role of economics and culture as well as the profit motive of manufacturers and plastic surgeons in the destruction of women's bodies.

4

Oh, You Beautiful Doll: Transforming the Self in American Culture

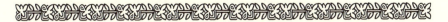

[E]veryone feels deformed. They want to look like something they're not.

—Hairdresser discussing women clients

Helen and Jay were sweethearts throughout high school in the late 1950s, living the dream for which their parents' sacrifices had prepared them. They were both college bound, he to be a basketball star, she to be with him. Then Helen got pregnant, and they "had to" get married. Plans for college were abandoned. Their marriage was punctuated by Jay's affairs, while Helen's guilt over "ruining his future" made her compliant. She tolerated the unaccounted for absences, the late nights, and the increasingly abusive verbal attacks. These were consistent with her traditional expectations about marriage and her sense of her own limitations, gilded by the responsibility she felt for her husband's dissatisfaction. As they aged, his criticism turned increasingly to her physical inadequacies and flaws, sagging breasts, stretch marks, and lumpy thighs, as he compared her with his other women, their younger, firmer bodies, their larger, fuller breasts.

Their relationship deteriorated; their interactions became perfunctory, he being demanding and accusatory, and she becoming more despairing and hopeless. The children were now grown, Helen was forty-seven, with no high school degree, a history of part-time clerical work, and feelings of inadequacy and failure. Their relationship sank to such a low level that she would draw his bath and iron his shirt when she knew he was going out with another woman, hating herself as she did so for her weakness and inadequacy, hating him for his arrogance and rejection. He chided her about her body, told her she could never expect him to stay home unless she "got bigger breasts, something for him to stay home for."

Despite his attacks, and despite her sense of failure and self-blame, Helen had never hated her body; her breasts were adequate, and she thought she "looked pretty good for her age." However, her husband cajoled and threatened, and feeling increasingly vulnerable and fearing the loss of her marriage, Helen finally agreed to have breast implants. She did not have a clear understanding of her decision: "I don't know what I was thinking—I just felt so guilty and thought he'd love me more. It was for him." Jay chose the plastic surgeon and accompanied her to the initial consultation. She remembers feeling dirty and inadequate as her husband discussed the size she should be with the surgeon. She felt invisible while the two men discussed volume, shape, and dimensions. She remembers her fear when, just before surgery, the doctor showed her larger implants than they had initially agreed to and proceeded to place them into her chest. She felt sick with dread, but soon had to deal with overwhelming physical problems; the stitches tore open before the wound healed, and she developed an infection in one breast. She was nauseated, and had severe headaches and flulike aches and pains. Her illness was accompanied by shame and embarrassment at her large breasts, and she bought bulky, loose clothing to conceal her unfamiliar body.

Silicone lumps began forming in her arms, her joints began to ache, and she began having night sweats and headaches and eventually wasn't well enough to hold down even a part-time job. She convinced Jay that she must have the implants out, and he reluctantly accompanied her to the out-of-town surgeon who agreed to remove them, while delaying payment until she received compensation from the settlement agreement that Dow Corning had made with plaintiff attorneys. The short plane trip was miserable, with Jay refusing to sit next to her, angry that she would want to "ruin her looks." Exhausted by the simple activities required for the trip, she arrived at the airport feeling like she had a severe flu. After the implants were removed, her strength gradually returned, and Helen, feeling wounded both physically and emotionally, at least knew that she would survive. When Jay finally left her, moving in with one of the several women he had been seeing, her relief overshadowed her pain, and she began the process of healing, both physically and emotionally, while adjusting to a chest that was deeply scarred and breasts that were now only hanging shreds of flesh.

Helen's experience, difficult as it was, was only one of the many painful stories I heard. I sat in her living room, drinking iced tea, and as we talked about children several years after her divorce, the edges of her memory softened. But our conversation also loosened the anger and pain she felt at her loss and mutilation. Our talk revealed the underlying cultural demands she responded to, the expectations she tried to meet, and her efforts to avoid abandonment and failure. Helen, like all women who have had breast implants, made her decision in a cultural context that limited the avenues by which she could remain valuable and that established her worth as intricately linked to the acceptability of her body.

Beauty images are products of longstanding patriarchal gender systems. Lowe's suggestion (1994:34) that in medieval and early modern Europe, the body and its deportment were the most obvious and controllable manifestations of that system, seems equally applicable to the situation of women with breast implants. Women became increasingly controlled by a gender system that included appropriation of the body and its appearance, and women lost not just their public voice in the process but their private voice as well. That is, their private voice could not be distinguished from the public voices that formed it. Their value as moral beings, always suspect, was represented by the body; the more the body could be shaped and controlled, the greater the possibility of controlling women's sensual, carnal nature, thus protecting men from temptation and maintaining the social order: "if she be a worthy woman of her body, all her faults are covered, and she can go with a high head" (from Philip of Navarre in the thirteenth century, in Lowe, 1994:24).

Lowe suggests that the commodification of women's bodies is based on distrust of women and on the assumption that women were in dire need of control because of their greater tendency toward sinfulness and their underlying wretchedness. The "feminine body became like a piece of clay to be formed, shaped and manipulated in an effort to save the weak female soul" (Lowe, 1994:23).

The forming and molding of women's bodies through such practices as genital mutilation are designed to control the female body and overcome its perceived imperfections, thereby diminishing the selfhood of the woman whose body it is. Such rituals are practical necessities if a girl is to survive in a society in which her only avenue to economic well-being is marriage to a man who demands such mutilation, not once, but often time and again, between each act of intercourse or each child (Daly, 1978). Those higher status young girls who had their feet bound not only demonstrated their family's worth, but also increased their chances of marrying well and prospering. Men who valued these mutilated women and the women themselves shared a common philosophy in which the gendered economic system and its attendant definitions of masculinity and femininity required the cutting, maiming, and scarring of women's bodies.

While the comparison may at first seem troubling, an analysis of the reasons women have breast implants reveals that the underlying issues are not so different from those motivating foot binding and genital mutilation. Almost 80 percent of women who have implants have them for cosmetic reasons (Stewart and Ross, 1996). While the women's justifications are cloaked in references to choice and self-esteem, deep down they believe they will be more attractive, more marketable, or simply more valuable if they have larger breasts. Self-esteem is indeed built within a cultural context, and women's self-esteem is essentially tied to body image (Tseëlon, 1995). In a society in which women have incorporated the "male gaze" and have learned to view themselves as objects to be assessed by men, their reflected self exists as a "spectacle . . . in permanent dissatisfaction with the visible self" (Tseëlon, 1995:76).

Women are likely to have implants at predictable times in their lives; when they are aging, recently divorced, or after having babies and finding their marriages faltering—that is, during times when their legitimacy as attractive, desirable women is being challenged. These women often report that they thought implants would either allow them to find a man or to keep one; such a goal allows economic well-being and in addition provides the women with a familiar and legitimate identity. To be one of those "not chosen" can have damaging economic and social consequences. Women in Somalia, Kenya, the Sudan, and Ethiopia insist that unless their daughters' genitals are cut and sewn no one will want them and they will have miserable lives spent without husband, children, or any means of support.

All of the interventions in women's bodies that have been mentioned in this book are designed to improve the woman through mutilation or surgical re-creation. All involve wounds that are deep and painful, requiring lengthy healing. All incorporate the risk of infection and illness and possibly death, either through blood loss, gangrene, or toxic chemicals spilled into a woman's body. All dramatically and permanently alter the woman's body, and all have enormous negative consequences for her emotional and physical well-being.

Clearly, women's social world and everyday experiences cannot be removed from cultural beliefs and definitions about their bodies and are intimately linked with economic and political power structures. If women had economic or political power, they would have no reason to alter their bodies; they would simply have it. But indeed, this is not so. Although American women are not likely to be killed by their husbands

for not bringing the promised dowry or bride price, the physical manip-
ulations and interventions they endure—from liposuction to facelifts to
waxes and peels—are a direct result of their relative economic powerlessness. Their position of political powerlessness is reflected in and re-
produced by their socialization.

Women are socialized to anticipate, and to be comfortable in, a political and economic environment in which they must rely on men for access to power and status. As Wolf (1991) suggests, women's distortion
of themselves into a spectacle acceptable to men divides them internally.
This process, when coupled with the negative emotions women associate
with their bodies (hence, themselves), leads to women's reflexive legitimation of oppression, a process by which they submit unconsciously to
subordination. Women's subordination relies on the internalization of
their inferiority and requires that they see themselves from men's dominant and dominating viewpoint.

Consistent with and supportive of this view is the reality of women's
economic experience. Although there are more women in the workplace
today than there were several decades ago, they still make just over
seventy cents to a man's dollar (Anderson, 1996). As Hochschild (1989)
says, they also put in a second shift, combining paid employment with
housework. Through the ghettoization of women's work, the disjunction
between home/family and the workplace, and the economic catastrophe
of divorce, women have severe economic disadvantages in this country
(Renzetti and Curran, 1992). Women, especially those with limited skills
or education and those who are socialized successfully to view themselves primarily in terms of their acceptability to others, may well learn
to make themselves valuable through manipulation of their bodies,
through a presentation of self that is artfully deceiving. In the insecure
environment occupied by women, they are always on display, on show,
scrutinized, examined, and judged—always psychologically alert to the
cues of others and to the success or failure of their performances.
Women's self-concept is influenced strongly by the norms and standards
that directly demand attractiveness and femininity, and much of their
time is spent in activities of self-surveillance, self-discipline, and self-
policing in order to meet those standards. As Spitzak points out, the
guard and prisoner coexist in women; "through internalization of male
gazes and values, women evaluate themselves as they are evaluated by
men" (1990:53). The absorbing rituals of self-improvement reaffirm the
gender structure and act as a key form of social control.

This internalization is transformative; it is the process through which
the "structures of society become the structures of our own conscious-
ness" (Bordo, 1989:53) and formal means of control are rendered irrele-

vant (Valentine, 1994:120). Efforts to look good, while expected of women, are at the same time ridiculed for their triviality and lack of substance. Thus, even if a woman succeeds in gaining a more beautiful body, a more desirable body that garners more attention and admiration, rarely is this achievement accompanied by real respect or social power (Jaggar and Rothenberg, 1993:459). On the other hand, if she "lets herself go," if she reveals who she is "beneath it all" by getting fat or getting old, she is condemned. Women are not just to remain attractive, but they are to camouflage the unacceptable essence. To present an attractive self is an indication of a commitment to a moral self, an agreement to overcome or make up for the flawed and potentially destructive self that abides in woman's dark inner life. The words of the monastic reformer Odo of Cluny are an extreme illustration of this view of woman's true nature as despicable, but they provide an historical standard against which women's moral progress can be measured:

> The beauty of a woman is only skin-deep. If men could see beneath the flesh and penetrate below the surface with eyes like the Beotian lynx, they would be nauseated just to look at women, for all this feminine charm is nothing but phlegm, blood, humors, gall. . . . We are all repelled to touch vomit and ordure even with our fingertips. How then can we ever want to embrace what is merely a sack of rottenness? (Warner, 1985; in Lowe, 1994:251)

If a woman cannot maintain her youth and beauty, at the very least she is expected to maintain her invisibility. The inherent paradox of femininity is that women are socially invisible while being physically and psychologically visible—always on stage, performing for an audience, camouflaging the unacceptable self, presenting an image that distracts from the essence. The actress is a perfect metaphor for women in Western culture—properly made up for presentation and appreciation, recognizing this as artifice, yet knowing that revelation of the self beneath the actor spoils the performance. Women's success is built on the early reviews, the acclaims or condemnations of critics whose judgments help shape women's futures.

For women the required focus on perfecting the imperfect body serves the social function of obscuring structural inequality and minimizing the possibility of concerted action to change the situation. If women are convinced that the only way to accomplish change in their lives is to change their bodies, from chin lifts to tummy tucks to breast implants, attention is deflected from inequalities of gender structure. Voices of social change are muffled, replaced by endless self-blame and self-recrimination. If women can be encouraged to focus on changing themselves, constantly working to overcome their imperfections through makeup, exercise, or surgery, if their view can be limited to their own body and its relative value vis-à-vis some unreachable standard, then women will not address the structural and economic realities that make it necessary to find their value through men in the first place. And if other women are the competition in this serious game, concerted social action based on shared social awareness is impossible. Helen, who introduces this chapter, is an excellent illustration of this turning against oneself and of competing with other women for male support, rather than analyzing her almost impossible position in terms of the economic and social positions she occupied in her marriage and in the larger society.

The control of women, then, need not be accomplished through force, although force against one woman, as Brownmiller (1975) claims, in the case of rape or sexual epithets, for example, is in fact a message to all women about boundaries and consequences. Control comes through scientific language, which has the advantage of appearing nonpolitical, presenting the body as an ideal type. This ideal is attainable through the woman's diligence, which requires ever more energy from the woman as she ages. And the outcome is necessarily failure; her efforts to conceal the deteriorating self become laughable and finally horrible.

The unadulterated images of the ideal body are leveling influences, quashing the personal desires and predilections of the individual so that "without overt coercion, persons abandon their cultural heritage, ethnic identity and customary approaches to constructing reality" (Murphy, 1994:73). This symbolic violence has a leveling effect on women—we become one. There is one rational ideal, and we are not it.

The knowledge base is asymmetrically arranged; the source of control is concealed and as such becomes inviolable; opposition is discredited. One can strive for perfection and court the ideal, but the ideal is embedded in an unchallengeable and omnipresent language of authority that the woman does not shape.

CULTURAL LESSONS

Cultural definitions of women and women's sexuality provide the backdrop against which we learn the demands of femininity and the expectations we are to fulfill in order to be rewarded in this culture. While it is clear that the economic and educational status of some women has changed, and dramatically so during the last several decades, the everyday reality for most women remains quite the same; their economic survival, especially if they have children, is tied to a man.

The literature on gender socialization is full of studies documenting the differences in gender socialization of males and females, and linking those differences to the familial and economic roles and statuses they are expected to find fulfilling (Best, 1983; Rheingold and Cook, 1975; Wolf, 1991). In storybooks, romantic songs, films, and novels, both males and females learn that men "do" while women "are" (Weitzman, 1974). A particularly ugly turn of this expectation that men do is the expansion of the term "do" to include men "doing" women. Beavis and Butt-head illustrate the hostility toward women's sexuality and being when they mistake the instruction to "do" a woman to mean rape her rather than kill her . . . a confusion that results in a barrel of laughs in their movie, *Beavis & Butt-head Do America*.

Differential expectations for boys and girls provide for the socialization of males into autonomy, decision making, and aggression and the parallel socialization of women into dependence, nurturance, and passivity. Not that these patterns are so extreme as to be visible in every interaction, but clearly the gender structure provides comfortable interactions and relationships based on gender inequalities reflected by the differential behavior of men and women.

Women are to find their value through their natural unfolding, through their acquiescence to the demands of nature, while men are expected to compete for scarce rewards, to overcome or conquer nature (Renzetti and Curran, 1992:344). Women learn to be relational selves while men learn to be solo selves; while women derive their value and their meaning through their relationships with others, both men and children, men are to find success through the ability to keep the demands of relationships from interfering with economic and political success. Because relationships are so central to women's self-image, feeling good about themselves is inextricably bound to being attractive to others. Being acceptable to others physically, given the close relationship between self-concept and body image, allows acceptance of the self (Tseëlon, 1995: 80). One can become oneself by engaging in the internal dialogue between self-meaning and the validation offered by others.

One of the most extreme early statements of women's reflected and derivative self is that offered by the psychologist, Erik Erikson (1968) in his assertion that the important developmental task for a female is to hold her self, her identity, in abeyance as she prepares to attract the man by whose name she will be known, the man who will rescue her from her emptiness and loneliness by filling the "inner space," allowing her the opportunity to bear his child (275–279). Today, while most theorists would not so blatantly posit such a reflected self for women, women's identity as an affiliate is supported by cultural imagery deeply embedded in the everyday taken-for-granted world in which we live. For women, intimacy and identity are to merge, allowing the woman to know herself as she is known—through her relationships with others. The expectations that shape women are subtle but powerful; they are reinforced in every aspect of culture and in the everyday interactions with parents, teachers, and peers. The fabric of expectations is densely woven; the messages of femininity are learned with one's first solid food, one's first step, one's first day in kindergarten (Anderson, 1966). As Sandra Bem concludes (1983), our lack of awareness of the profound gender demands of our culture is proof of their strength and pervasiveness.

From childhood through adulthood, women's experiences encourage them to derive their value and their deepest sense of self through their affiliations with others, through connectedness rather than separation, through merging rather than being apart. The marketing of Barbie and Ken provides a good example of the power of these socialization messages: Barbie reinforces girl's play that involves "dressing and grooming and acting out their future—going on a date, getting married," while Ken reinforces boy's play involving "competition and conflict, good guys vs. bad guys" (Lawson, 1989:C1; Renzetti and Curran, 1992).

In this culture, as in most others, a woman's opportunity to fulfill her role successfully, to be chosen as a wife and mother, depends heavily on her physical attractiveness. The interpersonal consequences of physical attractiveness are unequivocally stronger for women than for men; women are judged more critically for attractiveness and are rejected more severely when they lack it (Jackson, 1992, in Tseëlon, 1995:79). Women learn early and well that to be valued requires being desirable (Wolf, 1991; Wood, 1994). They also learn that overcoming faults and deficiencies, including the inevitable and natural consequences of aging, is a necessary, never-ending, increasingly difficult task. It is within this context that a woman's desire to have breast implants can be understood, as can women's efforts to achieve thinness and flawless skin—in short, perfection. Because such heavy emphasis is placed on how women look rather than on what they do, women make themselves and their appearance their project; women "do" themselves. Women put on their faces, do their makeup, their clothes, and their bodies, and in so doing, make up for their flaws.

Given this demand for the perfection of the ever-changing self which presents new challenges on a daily basis, it is not surprising that women evaluate themselves endlessly. It is even less surprising that they are merciless in these evaluations. Women find every flaw. Their images of themselves and their bodies are far more negative than those of men, who escape the body-as-self equation (Berscheid et al., 1973; Franzoi et al., 1989). Women are provided with unattainable models in the media and unrelenting demands to maintain control of their looks; they should "not let themselves go," and they necessarily fall short of perfection. A report by Miller et al. (1980) demonstrates the critical eye women acquire toward their bodies; 70 percent of the female college students questioned described themselves as being overweight, although only 39 percent could have been objectively described as such (Renzetti and Curran, 1992:345). Women's constant vigilance over their bodies leads to a pervasive vulnerability to messages of inadequacy and to demands for self-improvement. Because looks are their defining feature, women are required to maintain them in order to remain morally and socially legitimate (Mazur, 1986; Unger, 1985).

Not surprisingly, breasts are likely to be the focus of women's attempts to maintain and improve themselves, to achieve value. From an early age, women make efforts to alter the appearance of their breasts; little girls wear "training bras," and teenagers and adults wear "push up bras," perhaps the "Wonder Bra" or some variation thereof. These efforts reflect the strength of cultural messages, and they indicate their incorporation into everyday life.

Yet, women who attempt to negotiate an acceptable identity within the constraints of femininity through breast implants, often reacting to solicitation by plastic surgeons or encouragement by spouses or friends, are quite likely to be condemned as weak-willed, superficial, or vain when they become sick from silicone leakage or when their breast implants harden, migrate, or collapse. Their very incorporation of the dominant cultural messages about femininity leads to damaging decisions for which they are then individually condemned.

Breast implants can provide access to power through a relationship. They can enhance one's attractiveness and thus offer security, legitimacy of one's femininity, and sometimes employability. Indeed, as discussed later, those women who have few other attributes on which to draw for their identity, those who may feel most vulnerable to negative evaluations of their femininity, may be those most vulnerable to the appeal of this type of plastic surgery. Breast implant surgery is probably different from other types of plastic surgery, more central to the evaluation of self. Similarly, the loss of a breast is symbolically more powerful than, for example, the loss of an arm or leg, even though the lack of a limb may be far more visible and physically compromising.

The research on women who have had implants indicates a cluster of reasons they give for seeking breast augmentation; all the reasons center on the common theme of femininity (Beale et al., 1984; Kaslow and Becker, 1992). Kaslow and Becker suggest that women are attracted to

the idea of implants while in their thirties, "a time of fading attractiveness." This evaluation might strike the reader as absurd since it allows
for only ten years past one's teens for attractive womanhood, followed
by decades of increasingly devastating decline. Many of the women in
this study felt self-conscious about their small breasts or were otherwise
embarrassed by their bodies, and they anticipated that surgery would
increase their self-confidence and their feelings of femininity. Surgery,
some researchers say, represents an effort to "augment symbolically a
deficient sense of femininity, womanliness and attractiveness" (Birtchnell
et al., 1990:512).

Some authors (Goin and Goin, 1981) provide a more psychoanalytic
perspective on the reasons women have implants, dividing them roughly
into three groups: (1) those whose breasts represent the nurturing mother
they did not have or the mother within, and who are uncertain about
their femininity and feel incompletely realized as women; (2) those who
thought their breasts were adequate prior to pregnancy but found them
to be diminished after "postpartum involution"; and (3) the minority of
women who request implants for purposes of sexual exploitation or who
are exhibitionists. This last category might more accurately consist of
those who have implants for economic reasons, for example, dancers and
cocktail waitresses.

The reasons women give for having implants are situated in a cultural
context in which they are willing to change either through improving
their bodies (hence attractiveness, self-acceptance, and acceptance by others) or through reestablishing a past, more acceptable, body. Women
were either searching for self-enhancement, trying to recapture a previous, or fading self, or trying to "become normal" for the first time by
building a new self. Whether women wanted implants for augmentation,
for correction of a deformity (the definition of which is very subjective),
or for reconstruction, the reasons were situated in the woman's evaluation of self.

Those who had implants for augmentation frequently cited negative
feelings about themselves or a diminished sense of self as the motivation
for having implants. They thought that increased breast size would overcome or neutralize these negative feelings. Those who had breast implants for reconstruction after mastectomy often situated their decision
in a desire to "return to normal" or to "regain my old self," or to "just
feel like a woman." Sometimes the availability of implants and their
purported safety figured heavily in the decision to have a subcutaneous
mastectomy for fibrocystic disease. Those who had implants to correct a
deformity perceived a physical stigma that was damaging or potentially
damaging. They were convinced that correcting that deformity would

enhance their lives, resulting in a happier, more acceptable, more "normal" self.

Women are not victims, nor are they "cultural dopes" as Davis (1991: 30) points out; they are well aware of the cultural forces shaping their desires for breast implants. The fact that their decisions to have implants occur within a situational and cultural context that is powerful and often damaging does not mean that they are mindless puppets. It does mean, however, that in this instance, as in every other, one's self is a part of the social and cultural environment in which we live, and it cannot be understood apart from that environment.

The women interviewed for this book were similar to those studied by Birtchnell et al. who found that women who get implants are seeking to "symbolically boost their sense of femininity and womanliness" (1990: 509). Our research suggests, however, that breasts are not just symbolic of femininity and womanliness. Rather, they are deeply enmeshed with one's womanliness. Much of a woman's sense of herself and her evaluation of herself is based on her perception of the acceptability of her body, particularly her breasts. We found this connection to be prevalent and completely understandable given the thick cultural milieu surrounding breasts. Goin and Goin (1981) conclude that a large number of women seeking breast implants are uncertain about their femininity and feel "incompletely realized as a woman." However, our understanding is that femininity and womanliness are always, normally and predictably, a central part of every woman's identity. Gender is inescapably the primary determinant of women's lives, and it is here that women's evaluation of self is most vulnerable to doubt and attack. Goin and Goin also suggest that women's concern about their femininity stems from insufficient nurturing from their own mothers. Hence, the enlarged breast represents both the mother one didn't have and the mother within (1981: 201). Such an explanation medicalizes the choice to have implants, placing these women on the fringes of acceptable behavior and on the outskirts of normality. It hardly seems necessary to conjure psychoanalytic explanations for the central role played by breasts in women's lives. The cultural demand to pay attention to them is inescapable.

BODY IMAGE AND SELF-ESTEEM

How one's body map develops is not entirely clear, but scholars agree that children begin with a rather hazy sense of their bodies, which develops into a more complex, differentiated, and sharply delineated body concept as they mature (Fertig, 1993; Krueger, 1990). This process occurs as the individual interacts with others and the image of one's body is constructed through these conversations and observations. Others—for example, parents and other family members, peers, and eventually the media—provide mirrors for the growing child (Tiemersma, 1989), offering information and evaluation not only about specific parts of the body, but the body as a whole. Children, of course, learn not just from specific people, but from the culture as it is communicated through jokes, songs, advertisements, television, and magazines. They are bombarded with images of the good or beautiful as well as the ugly and unacceptable, and they become hypersensitive to these images. Their circle of awareness, extending from family to peers and then to a more generalized world, includes ample information for them to use in their assessment of their bodies and the comparative bodies of others and through that, their evaluation of themselves, the development of the "looking-glass self" (Cooley, 1902).

The picture or image one has of one's body includes not just a physical map but a judgment of that body as well (see Schilder, 1950; Thompson et al., 1990; Tiemersma, 1989). Particular parts of the body may be especially significant in this assessment, especially as we compare it and we learn that others compare it with an ideal type. There is a cultural standard of height, weight, and shape against which one's body image is formed. The image requires evaluation, and particular parts of the body such as breasts are central to that assessment, given the attention they receive in the media as well as in talk and observation. The person takes her body as an object, stands outside herself, and evaluates it based on her perceptions of how others would, or do, evaluate it. She subsequently acts toward her body based on these perceptions of others' evaluations.

For women the body is not a temple, nor is it a home for the self; rather, it stands for the self and is inseparable from it. Because women's value rests so strongly on the acceptability and attractiveness of their bodies, the self is intimately, inextricably intertwined with the body. A desire to change the body is a desire to change the self. To reconstruct the breasts is to reconstruct the self—to dismantle the old and to replace it with the new, the more acceptable, the more beautiful, the more feminine. Women who have breast implants are not simply trying to change their bodies. They are also attempting to shape a new self, to reconstruct the old self, to construct a body that displays a valued self.

Because the body is a presentation, a statement of self, and not simply another part of the self, reshaping it is undertaken within a larger enterprise of changing the self. What might otherwise seem like a dangerous and painful intervention becomes understandable as essential to this important work.

Women getting implants are not just getting better breasts; they are also getting a better self. Transformation of the self requires transformation of the body. So, a cost of $3,000 or so, a few days of discomfort, and the remote possibility of some physical problems seem a small price to pay when the result can be a new, acceptable, and valuable self. This is the situated reality of women who have breast implants. They aren't going from a cupsize "B" to a cupsize "C". Instead, they are going from unacceptable and ignored to valued and desired. And what woman is immune to the message that to be desired is to have value; to be wanted by someone else is an affirmation of self. If it takes the surgeon's scalpel and a few thousand dollars to transform undesirable to desirable, then it is without question money well spent.

Most of the women whose stories appear in this book had implants for cosmetic reasons or augmentation. They had implants to improve the self, to enhance self-image, or to overcome some perceived flaw that devalued the self. The situated realities of these women are not all the same. Each woman made a personal decision that was intricately linked to her own history and her own assessment of her situation.

CONVERSION—BEING SAVED

The stories women tell are illustrative of the path to the decision to have implants; it is usually a slow-moving, relatively undramatic path. Generally, the process is normalized by those friends, family members, and physicians who encourage the women to have the surgery. Every woman I spoke with thought that these implants were completely safe and would last a lifetime. Many of them, even those who were satisfied with the results after surgery, are now angry at themselves as well as at their doctors and the manufacturers for their illnesses and deformities. They have a difficult time reconciling their illness with the fact that they wanted the very things that they now think made them ill. The decision was not made in a vacuum, however. Instead it was part of a process, as we can tell from the women's narratives, during which women considered, reconsidered, and finally decided. Many of the women had long thought about implants but finally got them only when some significant change occurred in their lives. Others had given them little thought, but when presented with the opportunity gladly took it. Still other women only considered implants when they were presented as a solution to potential maiming and disfigurement.

It is necessary to understand a woman's decision to have implants within a context of decision making, situated within culture, and influenced by individual characteristics. It is perhaps useful to look at another type of decision making, one in which the self is also transformed, in order to understand this process. Women who get breast implants are similar to people who undergo other types of conversions of self, such as conversions to political or religious groups. In the conversion process, the old self is left behind and is replaced with a new one. The old, damaged, sinful self, the heathen self, is replaced by a pure, better, more valuable, more desirable self.

Generally in a conversion process, the potential converts are experiencing a number of conditions or situations that might be called "predisposing characteristics" (Lofland and Stark, 1965). Some of the feelings that might make a person receptive to significant life-altering change include a deep, enduring sense of dissatisfaction with the self and with one's life, or a discomfort with one's self and one's identity. For many of the women interviewed, this dissatisfaction centered on their appearance, specifically on their breasts, just as for many potential converts, there is an overwhelming sense of dissatisfaction with life and its lack of meaning and purpose. One woman exemplified this dissatisfaction, saying, "I always hated my breasts, and I thought I'd be a lot happier if I had bigger breasts." Another woman characterized her unhappiness as follows: "Since I was young, I always had a flat chest—my dad and brothers made fun of them, calling me a carpenter's friend, a flat. I knew I would feel better about my self if I had bigger breasts."

In some cases, this sense of dissatisfaction or dis-ease was accompanied by a crisis of some kind, such as a divorce or a husband's affair. As with conversion to a religious group, here the woman was in a state of crisis, built on a feeling of discomfort centered on her body. The opportunity to transform her body, hence herself and her value, was very seductive. Lofland and Stark (1965) suggest that those who are most vulnerable to the appeal of a group requiring significant sacrifice or alteration of identity are likely to have an orientation that allows for the philosophy of the group. In similar fashion, the women who saw breast implants as offering a brighter future and a better self were already likely to view body altering or other forms of "making up" the body as a reasonable or understandable idea.

In the process of conversion, individuals often experience what Lofland and Stark called "felt needs," desires to change their situation, to address dissatisfaction or disappointment. The women we interviewed were often looking for an answer to their flagging egos and deflated sense of self. They wanted a solution to their felt needs, and it was not difficult in this culture for these women to look at *themselves* as the problem that needed a solution. This tendency to look to themselves as the problem is consistent with the socialization of women which encourages a sense that women are "born wrong" as Schaef (1987) has said and have to "make up" for it throughout their lives. This is the feeling of being "the other," as de Beauvoir suggested (1952). Looking to ourselves is a natural outcome of the process that socializes women to be responsible for relationships, sexuality, and family, to placate, improve, or repair. Failure of the relationship, failure at sex, failure of the family is the woman's failure, a blemish on her self. Frequently, husbands encouraged the women to get implants in order to fix a bad relationship. Such was the case with Louise; her husband thought their sex life would be better if she "lost a few pounds and had bigger breasts."

In other cases, women feel such loss of value and attractiveness after the ravages of a divorce that they are willing to go to great lengths to make themselves more acceptable, to be saved. For many women, breast implants appear to be a solution to the problem of unattractiveness and the devalued self. Such women already believe alteration of the body is acceptable, even desirable.

Just being dissatisfied, even being dissatisfied and wanting bigger breasts, doesn't necessarily result in the decision to have implants. Rather, what occurs in the next stages of the process involves the cooperation and encouragement of other people in the woman's life. As already mentioned, the woman often knows someone who has implants and encourages her to get them too. This acquaintance may recount the positive experiences she has had as a result of implants—better self-image, more dates, clothes that fit better, more attention, a generally elevated sense of value. This person may introduce her to a plastic surgeon or even accompany her to the first appointment. In any case, it is often other women who encourage the woman to change herself through self-mutilation and pain, almost a self-abasement, to reemerge a new and better person.

In some instances, the "other" is a woman portrayed on television or described in magazines. Sometimes hearing a woman touting the benefits of implants on a talk show, or a celebrity with whom the woman identifies will lead her to a more serious consideration of breast implants as a solution to her problems.

At this stage, the woman encounters a plastic surgeon who redefines her problems as those that can be treated surgically. Her small breasts become the disease "hypomastia" or "micromastia," her breasts which are smaller after nursing become "postpartum involution," and her narrow chest becomes a "pigeon breast," all of which can be corrected through plastic surgery. This surgical entrepreneur reshapes her doubts about her self and her body into diseases that can be corrected by surgery. Once legitimated and validated as a person suffering a medical condition, the woman has more trouble accepting her old self and her old body. Now that she has a disease, now that she is a legitimate patient, her redefinition of self incorporates a new identity as a potentially large-breasted, happy, valuable woman. As one woman said, after she went home from the plastic surgeon's office, she and her husband had a celebratory drink and burned her padded bras in the fireplace—"out with the old, in with the new." This woman, like others, saw herself as transformed by implants, not only physically but spiritually; she would become a new person.

The conversion to "the new woman" is completed when she engages in a "bridge-burning act." In the case of religious converts, this is an act that cuts them off from the past and firmly places them in the present. In the case of women, it is surgery to provide breast implants. This act demarcates the old, inadequate self, the unsaved, from the new, worthy self, the moral self, the saved. Acclaim by others, recognition, and attention solidify her new identity. Most women who had implants were proud of the way they looked in clothes, and they were happily surprised by the remarks and appreciative looks they got from men. The male gaze followed them into the privacy of their bedrooms and bathrooms, comforting them with an acknowledgment of acceptability and self-worth.

After such an arduous process, and one that was so rewarding, it is small wonder that most women resist the possibility that their implants are making them sick, and are frightened by the prospect of being forced to return to the self they had so happily discarded.

5

A Nip, a Tuck, a Lift: Medicalizing Healthy Women

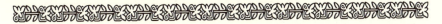

There is a substantial and enlarging body of medical information and opinion however, to the effect that these deformities (small breasts) are really a disease.

ASPRS, 1982

The medicalization of American life deserves significant attention because it is the umbrella under which the medicalization of women's bodies takes place. It establishes the environment in which surgical intervention to correct women's bodies to bring them into conformity with an ideal occurs. This process occurs not just with women's bodies, but with any number of phenomena that at one time were seen as either normal variations or were defined in other terms altogether, as sin, for example. In this chapter, many of the examples of medicalization are of behaviors that at one time were considered criminal or immoral or simply unruly, but that now, through the lobbying efforts of the medical establishment, have been transformed into medical problems.

Medicine has become the second largest industry in America. Over 350,000 physicians and over 5 million people are now employed in the medical field. Medical industries, including pharmaceutical, medical technology, and health insurance industries, are among the most profitable in our economy (Conrad and Schneider, 1992). Directly tied to these industries are the mental health professions, including the plethora of psychologists, counselors, marriage and family therapists, school counselors, drug and alcohol addiction therapists, and any number of lay therapists and other counselors with a variety (or deficit) of credentials. Hospitals and these mental health professions have cooperated in the development of inpatient and outpatient programs, underwritten by the insurance companies, often owned by the hospitals. Most recently, they have focused on various addictive behaviors, but were preceded in the recent past by programs for obesity and anorexia and other eating disorders, in addition to the more traditional disorders.

As long as a person has a good medical insurance program, time, and the willingness to be hospitalized or to become an outpatient, she or he will find a welcoming hospital or therapist. The fact that there is no indication that these hospitals successfully treat or "cure" the illnesses to which they devote themselves, or that therapy is effective, does not seem to diminish the reliance on them. Nor does it dampen the insurance companies' enthusiasm for treatment within the limits of the policy.

Women who have breast implants are not seeking hospitalization for long-term treatment, but they are being transformed into patients as their bodies are reinterpreted as diseased. Their experience is part of the underlying eagerness to redefine variation as illness and to proffer a medical cure for all manner of social, personal, emotional, and interactional ills.

Medicalization, as a process, includes the increasing reliance not just on particular medical explanations for individual disease, but on the expansion of the definition of medical to include emotional problems and problems in everyday living. Rather than being defined as the human condition or interactional problems, or simply part of the expected process of growing up and growing old, our difficulties have become redefined as mental and emotional problems, to be treated through therapy or drugs or some combination thereof.

The medical industry's enormous growth during this century reflects both the increasing emphasis on progress through science and the successful interest group activity of medical associations and their affiliates. Concern about a doctor shortage in the United States during the 1950s and 1960s led to increased federal funding of medical schools between 1965 and 1980, resulting in an increase not only in the number of doctors, but also in the number of medical specializations. With the ever-increasing rise in the prestige of scientists and physicians, other professions adopted the medical model in their explanations of events. Problems such as excessive drinking, obnoxious or inappropriate behavior, recalcitrance or incorrigibility which in the past were viewed as a result of individual will or lack thereof, were now transformed into sicknesses, syndromes, and diseases by the medical and allied professions (Conrad and Schneider, 1992).

Nowhere is the medicalization of social phenomena more clearly illustrated than in the transformation of "acting out" to attention deficit disorder. This has meant a multimillion dollar windfall to psychologists, counselors, psychiatrists, pharmaceutical companies, and family physicians, not to mention school districts who rely on federal and state-funded programs for special education.

Another obvious example is the transformation of incest from a sin to a sickness. Whereas father-daughter incest was at one time seen as a reprehensible crime, a felony offense, the work of pop therapists such as Giaretto readily transformed it into a disease, symptomized most clearly by "inappropriate sexual object choice" and treatable through therapy (Giaretto, 1980). This therapeutic treatment was not directed solely at the perpetrators, whom therapists often referred to affectionately as "my dads." It also extended to the whole family, the daughter and mother being required to acknowledge their important role in the dysfunctional family (Stewart, 1991).

The proliferation of "addictions"—love addictions, drug addictions, alcohol addictions, shopping addictions, and the like—in the seventies and eighties was illustrated by the work of Woititz, 1983; Wegscheider-Cruse, 1981; Subby and Friel, 1984; and Beattie, 1987 on co-dependence and culminated with the broadest definition available offered by Anne Wilson Schaef in *When Society Becomes an Addict*. This emphasis on addictions shows the increasing unwillingness to attend to structural, political, and economic explanations for social problems, and the countervailing tendency to "fix" the person. This tendency is very consistent with the breast implant phenomenon.

Co-dependence, a term that is almost devoid of meaning but is useful for its breadth and ease of applicability, is an intriguing area to analyze because it so clearly illustrates the emergence of medicalization and sets the stage for the medicalization of women. While no valid research suggests the actual existence of such a phenomenon that can be reliably separated from other characteristics, therapists and counselors have embraced it as an explanation for everything from wife beating to alcoholism. The alcoholic, in fact, (e.g., Cermack, 1986) results from the co-dependent behavior of the spouse. This recent finding duplicates years of common knowledge espoused in bars and coffee shops across America that "she drove him to drink" or "anyone married to that woman would drink."

The abused wife is no longer defined as masochistic, except in some rigidly orthodox psychiatric circles; instead, she is deemed co-dependent. Rather than look to the patriarchal system, definitions of masculinity and femininity, and economic and political realities faced by these women, for an explanation we turn to their socialization into victim roles and their individual psychopathologies. Treatment in all of these cases focuses on building self-esteem. Women are especially prone to lack this quality in the current parlance, which individualizes characteristics and avoids situating women in the context of a society in which they are devalued. It is within this framework that breast implants are suggested as the surgical solution to low self-esteem.

Reliance on individual or familial dysfunctions as the cause of social problems, whether we are discussing criminality, academic failure, problem drinking, gambling, or sexual behavior, has dominated the previous two decades. Note, for example, the Menendez brothers who almost escaped punishment for murdering their parents because the jury was convinced that they had been abused as children, or the Polly Klaas case in which her monstrous killer's lifetime of crime was used to demonstrate not the failure of the justice system or his heinous behavior, but his pattern of illness resulting from damage to his self-image and personality as a result of an abusive childhood.

Child abuse, rape, domestic battery—all have been pulled into the quicksand of medicalization. The psychological literature, including the enormously powerful *Diagnostic Statistical Manual*, finds individual psychosis or neurosis at the base of all such problems, rather than such factors as economics, socialization, or simply, pervasive sexism and ageism. Rape, for example, is explained not only in terms of the rapist's personality but also in terms of the characteristics of the victim. Such journals as *Victimology* are devoted to studies of characteristics of the old, the infirm, the dispossessed, the murdered, or the assaulted which predictably result in their victimization. Scully and Marolla (1993) demonstrate the predictability of not only rape but also of the justifications and excuses offered for it by rapists as reflections of social constructions of reality. While such authors as Russell (1982) and Dworkin (1974) illustrate the destructive impact of woman hating and "rape culture," therapists are busy looking for intrapsychic clues for this relatively ordinary behavior. The same is true for attention deficit disorder; rather than look at the increasing pressures and incapabilities of stressed families, or the disorganization of the educational institutions, focus is turned to a serotonin problem in the brain of the acting-out child (Conrad and Schneider, 1992). The complex and deeply rooted economic and social problems that are endemic to many educational institutions and the communities they serve are thereby ignored or minimized. They may be contributory, but certainly they are not primary causes according to the many psychologists, teachers, and parents who have built their lives around the power of such a disorder.

The medicalization of women's bodies takes place within a context that first assesses their worth in terms of their bodies and then sees that worth as inadequate or declining, and demands that women do something about it by changing themselves. Rather than acting toward the world, changing structures, and political and economic realities, the same culture that defines women as so lacking provides the solution—change the self. This process, resulting in enormous physical and emotional damage to women, though not improving their economic and social status, is accomplished through the interface of cultural definitions of imperfection, demands for self-improvement, and the medicalization of women's bodies. Women are transformed into patients, seeking medical care to correct a deformed or inadequate self.

Through medicalization of their bodies, women are encouraged to bring themselves into conformity with a cultural ideal, to embrace the internal and external intrusions on their bodies in order to reap the benefits of attractiveness or even acceptability. This focus on the inadequacy of the self and the rewards of changing that self provides profits for the cosmetics and beauty industry, and puts riches in the pockets of the plastic surgeon. Cosmetic surgery is a popular and acceptable way of improving upon nature, often described by those who have undergone it as a normal and natural pursuit, akin to buying make-up or having their hair done (Dull and West, 1991; Tseëlon, 1995). Over 750,000 women a year in the United States undergo some sort of cosmetic surgery, resulting in a $450 million per year business (Regush, 1992:22).

Plastic surgery is the most rapidly growing speciality in medicine. Between 1965 and 1989, the number of physicians who considered themselves to be plastic surgeons increased fourfold, over twice the rate of physicians as a whole. Projected growth in the number of plastic surgeons for the year 2000 is 1100% as compared to a projected 44% increase in the general population (Porterfield, 1983; Zones, 1992).

Cultural messages that condemn women as imperfect, while simultaneously demanding that they change, improve, or perfect themselves, increase women's vulnerability to the medicalization of their bodies. And among plastic surgeons, the enthusiasm for using the scalpel to achieve perfection is great. As one Texas plastic surgeon opined, "The Texas woman is a combination of many things, not the least of which is a surgeon's scalpel" (Regush, 1992:96). Only about 64% of the 4492 physicians in the U.S. who identified plastic surgery as their main activity were board certified in 1989 (Zones, 1992). "In most states, any certified general surgery specialist may perform cosmetic surgery and in some states, any licensed physician may do so" (Zones, 1992). Some physicians learn their procedures at weekend workshops sponsored by specialty associations such as the American Society of Plastic and Reconstructive Surgeons. The debate within the medical profession over this certification continues, with some seeing certification as an effort to limit competition and others as an indication of expertise. For now, it results in an abundance of physicians who can be called upon to perform cosmetic surgeries, including breast augmentation. Strategies to increase the demand for cosmetic surgery include promoting its benefits through education and advertising, providing easy financing and minimizing its potential ill-effects.

Cosmetic surgery is, of course, only one of the more recent medical interventions in women's bodies which have proven a mother lode for manipulation, intervention, and control. Physicians, in any number of ways, seek to pathologize women's bodies, transforming natural processes into medical problems. Women's reproductive processes have long been a particularly attractive region for the expansion of medical turf, resulting in the medicalization of menstruation, pregnancy, childbirth, lactation, and menopause. Moving beyond functions of women's bodies that have been medicalized, such as childbirth and menopause, with cosmetic surgery, including breast implants, normal body variations are transformed into "objectively" problematic conditions and the aesthetic realm becomes legitimate terrain for expansion of medical authority (Dull and West, 1991; Reissman, 1983). The creation of these new disease categories (e.g., hypoplasia, hypomastia, micromastia, involutional atrophy, ptosis, postpartum atrophy) confirms the notion of the female body as a product, the packaging of which assures its salability.

The process of medical professionalization, which itself reflects dominant cultural definitions of woman's value (Reissman, 1983; Wood, 1994), encourages the view that women's bodies require intervention if they are to be acceptable. "Beauty for women is a temporary state which only underlines the fact that their value is measured in how well they succeed in the role of a spectacle" (Tseëlon, 1995:89). Women, readily transformed into patients by the medical establishment, are assumed to be less reasonable than men and more likely to exhibit emotional rather than physical problems. So, this tendency to medicalize women expands the numbers while at the same time denying the seriousness of their illnesses. Women's cooperation in this process both emerges from and reinforces their subordination.

Women are securely locked within a lifelong "medical gaze," as Foucault (1973) suggests, and their natural, everyday life experiences are transformed into illnesses or disabilities. Even an acknowledgment of women's reproductive function, such as time off from work for childbirth and the early weeks of recovery and caring for the infant, is traditionally defined as "disability leave." Thus, the perfectly natural human female experience of pregnancy and childbirth is transformed into a sickness. Both the doctors and pharmaceutical companies have come to the rescue of premenstrual, menstrual, and menopausal women (and all women teetering on the edge of one of these conditions) victimized by their wild and raging hormones. The natural processes of women's lives have increasingly come under the control of various medical specialists, resulting in unnecessary medical treatment and surgical intervention.

When they are still girls, women learn that they cannot trust their own bodies and that, in fact, their bodies are not truly their own. In high school or even earlier, they become aware that their bodies can be the subjects of male aggression, when their appearance, behavior, or dress attracts male attention. Thus, at a very early age, women learn to dissociate the self from the body, and realize that the body is not fully theirs; at the same time, they begin to realize that their value is assessed in terms of that very body. While they must treat it as an object and have it evaluated as an object, they do not have the freedom to do with it what they will—the consequences are too severe. Their alienation from their body is overwhelming.

Women also learn, as they begin to menstruate, that their bodies are unclean, contaminated, even polluted. Women in the United States may not be sent to the huts to bleed, but drugstore shelves are lined with deodorant tampons, a dizzying array of pads, wipes, special douches, and other products to decrease the supposed natural offensiveness of the female body. Concern about PMS and related emotional and physical discomforts during "that time of month" accompany women into relationships, the workplace, and in competition for political office. Women are expected to camouflage with "feminine hygiene products," which have nothing to do with hygiene, the odors they are suspected of producing, which are presented as offensive, and destructive to their relationships and jobs.

While the female body is essentially unacceptable and dangerous, it is also precious and in need of protection. Women are supposed to guard their body and restrict their behavior, and at the same time prepare and present it to be admired and desired by their male audience. Biologists and anthropologists have lent scholarly credence to these ideas by suggesting that women's manipulaton of their bodies over the centuries simply reflects the genetic encoding that draws males during the reproductive years to the most physically attractive females in order to perpetuate the healthy human race.

As women have children and leave their childbearing years, their value plummets. Plastic surgery becomes the most sought-after surgery for women during this time, enabling them to postpone the decline and maintain or enhance value. In today's economic marketplace, with its high incidence of divorce, with women's earning power comparatively low, and with little hope for change in the near future, women are understandably vulnerable to appeals for improving their looks in order to remain competitive. Women may recognize the inequity of the economic system and may, in their more abstract discussions with others, deride the men who leave their spouses of twenty years for trophy wives or to begin their second-tier marriages. Nevertheless, women in their daily decisions respond to the demands of the moment. In the moment, the goal is to reestablish the self as valuable, and if this means a facelift, breast lift, tummy tuck, liposuction, or any number of other small or more dramatic interventions, so be it. The struggle to retain the outward self, to protect the value of the inner self, and to avoid the failure of aging are efforts to avoid being discredited. These efforts propel women toward anything that will erase the signs that the self has fallen into disrepair or disrepute.

Women's awareness of self through their awareness of male evaluation serves to control women through the negative imagery of imperfection. Plastic surgery is built on this imagery, and its promise to improve women by shaping them into acceptable form sustains their reliance on their bodies for their value and acts as a control agent, reinforcing female dependency and self-degradation. This more subtle form of control is a spinoff from the more blatant ways in which physicians have supported male control over women's lives for over one hundred and fifty years. Over the generations doctors have succeeded in controlling women's lives by advising that women be kept out of universities because mental function would interfere with the more essential reproductive function; leading the fight against birth control and to make abortion illegal; and defining women's natural biological processes as medical diseases (Ehrenreich and English, 1986; Fausto-Sterling, 1985; Wood, 1994).

This effort to control the female body has reinforced cultural definitions of appropriate femininity and reflects the desire to maintain women in their position so that men can fulfill their own goals. It is not a conspiracy by any means; rather, it is a straightforward reflection of the assumptions about everyday life. Those persons who hold positions of power in what Bernstein (*Blum v. Merrell Dow*, 1996) has called the medical-industrial complex emerge from the same social world as do the rest of us, carrying with them the same cultural belief systems. Hence, their orientation to women and to women's bodies can be expected to deviate little from that of the rest of the population. Given the financial incentive, they can draw on everyday popular cultural imagery in their efforts to increase their clientele, even if they do not wholeheartedly embrace it. Indeed, women are surrounded by the unattainable image of perfection in popular culture presented through the media, which consistently and tirelessly remind them of their imperfection and consequent lack of worth.

In their effort to achieve even a temporarily positive evaluation of the self, women seek breast implants. The constant vigilance required to overcome the stigma of the female body, a demand that divides the self against itself, has provided fertile soil for the growth of the breast implant industry. Breast augmentation offers a new area to be mined by the medical claimsmakers, with painful social and economic consequences. Among these claimsmakers are entrepreneurial plastic surgeons who are available to contour, enhance, augment, and erase, as well as their professional associations which provide political support, funding, and lobbying, and manufacturers who provide products and surgical instruments. Affiliated personnel also involved in the sale and construction of the acceptable female form include secretaries, nurses, attendants, janitors, hospital staff, anesthesiologists, insurance clerks, and producers of the related necessary products.

Breast implants are a lucrative form of plastic surgery, with between 120,000–150,000 women in the United States having breast implants each year prior to their restriction (Japenga, 1993; Zones, 1992). Nearly 1 million women in this country have had implants; the vast majority have done so for purely cosmetic purposes.

The search for third-party payments and the desire to legitimize the plastic surgery medical specialty may have contributed to the efforts to define women's small breasts as a medical problem. Reissman (1983) suggests that medicalization is likely to occur whenever physicians can serve the broader interests of their patients, while at the same time enhancing their own political and economic interests. It is probably predictable that the ASPRS has defined the bodies of millions of women in this country as deformed and has suggested surgical intervention to correct this devastating deformity. In this way, the number of women who can be legitimate patients has been vastly increased:

There is a common misconception that the enlargement of the female breast is not necessary for maintenance of health or treatment of disease. There is a substantial and enlarging body of medical information and opinion however, to the effect that *these deformities [small breasts]* are really a disease which in most patients results in feelings of inadequacy, lack of self-confidence, distortion of body image and a total lack of well-being due to a lack of self-perceived femininity. The enlargement of the under-developed female breast is, therefore, often very necessary to insure an improved quality of life for the patient. (ASPRS quoted in Zones, 1992:236; author's emphasis)

When we examine this claim, several questions arise: Is this "substantial and enlarging body of medical information and opinion" mostly "information" or mostly "opinion"? And if it is information, is it based on studies done by reputable persons without bias, following strict guidelines for the production of scientific evidence? Where is the substantiation for the lack of self-confidence and well-being? Is it conjecture, empathy, or data? And how do we judge "underdeveloped"—by objective or by purely subjective standards? How might we establish objective standards for "underdeveloped" in any case? And whose standards should be applied—the woman's, her doctor's, or her husband's? When did the woman become transformed into the patient—when she made the appointment? when she inquired about implants? when she received the implants?

A careful literature review reveals that the reports of "total lack of well-being" are to be found in the professional journals in the field of plastic surgery. The studies that provide the background for these conclusions are conducted by plastic surgeons who have an obvious self-interest in the results (Zones, 1992). Furthermore, studies on the relationship between implants and psychological well-being are reported in journals published by the ASPRS and related specialties and are almost exclusively of women who had implants after mastectomy. One would expect them to feel better about having breasts than not having them, for a variety of reasons, including feeling whole, like a woman, or like themselves, just as they report.

Given the patient base on which these studies are conducted, it is hardly surprising that most of the research concludes that breast augmentation (usually for reconstruction after mastectomy) is psychologically beneficial to the patient and that the surgery enhances her feelings of self-worth and self-esteem. Indeed, the women we interviewed often reported being pleasantly surprised, even thrilled, with the results, at least at first. Women who seek breast implants for reasons other than reconstruction after mastectomy usually do so specifically to improve their self-esteem or feelings of femininity. Thus, it is no surprise that once they have the long-dreamed-of breasts, they feel more feminine and their self-esteem increases.

Very few studies have been done on the psychological or social characteristics of women who have breast implants; most such studies involve women who have had mastectomies. Between 1980 and 1991, no articles on this topic appeared in any American journal; almost all of them were published in either British or Scandinavian journals (Kaslow and Becker, 1992:469). Birtchnell and colleagues (1990) conclude that women want implants because their feelings about themselves as women, mothers, and lovers are tied to their breasts. Augmentation increases their feelings of femininity and therefore "symbolically augment(s) a deficient sense of femininity, womanliness, and attractiveness" (12). This, of course, may be true, but does it distinguish women who have implants from other women who do not, or from women who have other sorts of plastic surgery? The authors, while implying a particular deficiency among these women, thus supporting a sickness model, provide no evidence that this is particularly true of women with implants. Other researchers have concluded that women who seek implants (and those who seek lipectomy) suffer from a wide range of "psychopathologies, ranging from anorgasmy (100%) to inferiority complex, anxiety, sadness, insomnia, and bulimia" (Birtchnell et al., 1990).

An inferiority complex and oversensitivity to criticism were so debilitating to 93 percent of the patients in the Birtchnell study that they were unable to participate in social activities or to enjoy sexual relations. Some were even suicidal. These women clearly had a discredited self, which they were attempting to overcome through medical correction. As mentioned earlier, some researchers concluded that women wanted implants because they were uncertain about their femininity and felt "incompletely realized as a woman," a condition they suggested (with no support) stemmed from insufficient nurturing from their own mothers. This reader was relieved at least to see no reference to the inner or wounded child in such research, something that one could easily imagine given the symbolic connection of breasts with nurturing. All of these psychological explanations for getting implants hardly seem necessary. What may be of more interest is why some women get breast implants while others opt for facelifts or some variation thereof.

Based on our interviews and questionnaires, we learned that most of these women were from service and clerical occupations, and had relatively limited educational achievements and job opportunities. Compared with women who have other forms of cosmetic surgery, these women are less well-educated and less prosperous. While women who choose other types of plastic surgery are likely to be married to professional men or to be professionals themselves, women who had breast implants were more likely to come from blue-collar or working-class backgrounds. Women who are professionals tend to rely more on fitness classes and facelifts to keep their jobs and their men. Those who are more likely to rely on their breasts embrace a definition of worth and value that is more related to the body, at least to their breasts, than to their faces. Only a couple of the women whose records we viewed had any other sort of facial cosmetic surgery. Do these two types of improvement appeal to entirely different types of women? Is this class related? occupationally related? We aren't sure at present, but we do know that the figures and findings about cosmetic surgery in general should not simply be applied to women who have breast implants for cosmetic purposes.

ASPRS AND WOMEN'S INTERESTS

Given their keen interest in the implant market, the ASPRS has heavily lobbied the FDA to keep implants on the market, in one case flying women to the FDA hearings in Washington, D.C., from all over the country to testify about their need for these devices. The ASPRS also collected $1,050 from each of its 3,700 members during 1970 to step up its lobbying efforts and to counteract the growing negative publicity about breast implants. Plastic surgeons have cooperated with manufacturers in the production and testing of these devices and have ignored warnings about their potential danger. They often see such warnings as the work of litigation-mad attorneys and hysterical women, and so continue to place implants in women's bodies with absolutely no assurance of their safety (U.S. Congress, 1993). Plastic surgeons, through the ASPRS, have continued their lobbying efforts to keep silicone implants on the market, and also to dramatically alter the FDA requirements on informed consent and thereby expand the audience to whom implants can still be legally given. Dr. Marcia Angell (1992), currently Executive Editor of the *New England Journal of Medicine* and author of *Science on Trial*, has supported the ASPRS's claims. She reports that the subjective benefits of breast implants are substantial, and since it is the FDA's responsibility to assess the risk-benefit ratio rather than to determine safety, policymakers should consider the subjective benefit to women.

The ASPRS has had some success in watering down warnings about the possible debilitating effects of implants. As noted earlier, the association was able to significantly change the warnings about capsular contracture, misrepresenting the frequency of its occurrence to be about 10 percent of the cases, whereas other research indicates a contracture rate of about 40 percent (U.S. Congress, 1993). Some of their efforts to

change the wording of the "informed consent forms" also resulted in weakening the warnings about silicone gel migration, minimizing the dangers of breastfeeding, and dismissing any possible relationship between implants and breast cancer. ASPRS lobbying was also effective in changing the word "cancer" to the word "lesion" in information provided by the FDA. The ASPRS also lobbied to change the FDA's warning about closed capsulotomies. Because women presumably become hysterical or are easily confused, the ASPRS and the American Medical Association were concerned that severe warnings included in the informed consent forms would cause "unnecessary concern in a woman whose decision has already been made" (U.S. Congress, 1993:39).

Conrad and Schneider (1992) characterize the "dark side" of medicalization as including domination by experts, individualization of social problems, dislocation of responsibility, and decontextualization of social problems. The breast implant tragedy certainly illustrates this dark side. From Conrad and Schneider's perspective, medicalization serves as an agent of social control, determining the narrow range of "normal" and providing treatment for those who dare to deviate. When looking at the dark side of medicalization, it is important to include the physical and emotional damage done to those whose bodies have been the locus of medical intervention. Current litigation aimed at compensating women for damages suffered as a result of implants only begins to acknowledge this reality. The agreement reached in the now defunct global settlement was a small step toward remunerating the women for their damages.

But the women in our study know that they will never regain their health and that no amount of money will compensate them for this loss. Furthermore, the extent of the damage done by implants is still unknown. Approximately 75 percent of women in America who had implants had them between 1980 and 1990, even though implants had been on the market since 1964. Yet, it generally takes between five and seven years, often longer, for symptoms to emerge. This means that a large number of implanted women may not develop difficulties until 1997 and beyond. In addition, current research is starting to reveal more of the connections between silicone and related diseases, including problems in children who were breast fed by implanted women (Levine and Ilowite, 1994; Vasey and Feldstein, 1993).

Medicalization is potentially devastating to women. Women find themselves caught in a vicious trap; on the one hand, their worth is tied to their bodies, and on the other hand, they are treated despicably when their efforts to improve those bodies fail. In the process of writing this book, one of the most predictable responses from people, men and

women alike, was a mocking dismissal of the women who got implants as stupid, vain or worthless. This reaction came from the same people who clearly understand the paramount importance of looks for success and happiness in American culture.

6

Women's Bodies, Women's Worth

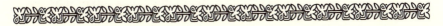

I'd just gone through a divorce, was alone with my kids, turning forty and somehow thought if I looked like Marilyn Monroe, I'd feel better about myself.

—Breast implant recipient

The controversy over breast implants has become part of our national debate, linked closely to the political discourse about tort reform and individual and corporate responsibility. While the press has dutifully, albeit superficially, reported the continuing negotiations between the major manufacturers and the litigants' representatives, and has covered the global settlement and its demise, the lives of the women who have suffered from the implants have generally gone unnoticed. Except for two-minute clips on talk shows and some brief interviews with a few individuals on news programs, the victims and their families are socially invisible. Indeed, to some extent this is of their own choosing, for many are embarrassed or exhausted by their condition. To a large extent this human face has been overlooked through all the attention given to the efforts of the AMA and ASPRS to defend implants and the efforts of the manufacturers to protect themselves from liability.

Yet a good deal of research has been conducted and published, much of it extremely controversial. Numerous medical journals have given attention to implants. Our own review of the literature reveals hundreds of articles on silicone gel and gel-filled implants and related materials. In addition, popular magazines as well as law journals and academic journals have published articles on this topic. In all of this research however, women have been examined as objects—specimen-objects in much of the medical research, plaintiff-objects in the legal research, and client-objects in psychological research. Little of the literature speaks to the lived reality of these women: their motivations, the impact of implants on their lives, the consequences of silicone-related problems. This chapter presents this lived reality and describes the efforts of these women to overcome or avoid a devalued status and to achieve a new physical and moral self.

Women evaluate their breasts against a standard of perfection that is unattainable; it is no surprise that they want to perfect their breasts, enlarging, lifting, shaping. Women are awash in cultural images of per-fect bodies and beautiful breasts and know full well whether they meas-ure up. Nowhere is this more clear than for a woman who has had a mastectomy. It's taken for granted that she will want implants to "nor-malize" her body; this procedure is often presented as the last stage of mastectomy surgery.

Most women who have implants have healthy but small breasts, or breasts that are not what they were twenty years ago. While some women simply want bigger breasts, most capture their dissatisfaction by adopting a medical label such as postpartum atrophy.

The reasons women want implants in the first place differ dramatically. Some women are trying to overcome what they have begun to see as a physical defect (small breasts, droopy breasts, inverted or misplaced nip-ples, and the like), others are trying to improve themselves and their lives, and still others are trying to return to normal after childbirth or after mas-tectomy. We'll look at these motivations separately because the stories they entail are different and the responses on the part of the women and of others to their implants can be expected to be quite different. At the same time, they share many similarities. All women with implants are respond-ing to a culturally consistent definition of femininity and are making up for some perceived or perceptible flaw or inadequacy. This may be a prob-lem of identity, a problem related to an economic condition, or a problem of the physical body. Furthermore, the women are often held responsible for the pain and damage they experience as a result of the implant, blamed for being vain and for trying to improve on what God has given them, or viewed as simply taking risks they now have to live with, which is a par-ticularly egregious form of victim-blaming.

THE WOMEN

Most of the women in our study had implants because they didn't like the way their breasts looked, primarily because they were too small. Of the sixty-three women who returned questionnaires to us, 68 percent had implants for this reason. Of these, about 20 percent added that they had "postpartum atrophy," which indicated that their breasts had become more flaccid or smaller after nursing. About that same number said they had a "congenital deformity"—for example, an undeveloped breast, breasts of very different shapes, nipples that were misplaced or inverted, or breasts that were not evenly placed. A smaller proportion (about 30 percent) had implants after mastectomy; most of these were as a result of mastectomy following fibrocystic disease and the remainder were after mastectomy for breast cancer.

Previous research suggests that women who have implants for breast reconstruction after mastectomy are relatively well educated (61 percent at least completed high school), and about the same number (63 percent) were employed full or part time (Rowland et al., 1993). Most of the women in Rowland's study were upper middle class, white (89 percent) and married (77 percent), and a large number were Catholic (45 percent). This study exemplifies the types of studies that are available. They are generally based on one patient base, and so are not necessarily representative (i.e., note that 45 percent of Rowland's subjects were Catholic). Since they are not comparative, we don't know how these women differ from those who had mastectomy but decided not to have reconstructions after their operation. Increasing numbers of women do, however, choose reconstruction, partly because less intrusive surgeries are now conducted with breast cancer and partly because of the ready availability of saline implants.

In another study of women who had implants for reconstruction after mastectomy (Winer et al., 1993), the women were on average between forty and fifty-nine years of age, almost all were white (2 percent nonwhite), 64 percent were employed, and the majority were Protestant. This sample does appear to be especially well-educated; 37 percent had a college degree or had done postgraduate work, while 30 percent had a high school diploma or less. Both the Rowland and Winer studies were based on particular samples of women in separate surgery practices in which the researcher attempted to work up a description of the women who were likely to obtain implants after mastectomy. The women included in the study may be influenced by the area of the country, the location of the practice, and the social characteristics of the population in that particular area.

Studies of women who have had implants for cosmetic purposes, primarily for augmentation, suggest that these women are somewhat younger than those having them for reconstruction. Kaslow and Becker (1992) found that 87 percent of the thirty-two women in their Palm

Beach, California sample were between twenty-five and forty-four years of age, with about 56 percent in their thirties. These women were also more likely to be high school graduates (41 percent) than college graduates (19 percent) or to have some college (19 percent). In our sample, 18 percent had less than a high school degree, 29 percent had graduated from high school, another 37 percent had some college or technical training, and 16 percent had a college degree or more education. These are the characteristics of our sample and do not necessarily represent all of the women who had implants.

The women in our sample were likely to be employed, but there were no high-status professionals in this group. Although a large majority are currently unemployed owing to their illness and many are on disability, those who are employed are likely to work in service or clerical positions. The usual occupations of these women reflects women's occupational status more generally, except that because the study included a number of women from Nevada, 12 percent of the respondents were casino workers. In addition to those in service and clerical positions (55 percent), 18 percent were professionals and 13 percent were homemakers.

In our study, 60 percent of the women were married, with 32 percent being divorced. Only two were single, never married, and marital status data were missing for the remainder. Most of the women had children, with their median age at the birth of their first child being 19½. Eighty-four percent of the sample had their first child while they were under twenty-five, and 64 percent of these were under twenty-one when they first gave birth, a pattern not unique to women with breast implants.

The median current age of the women in our study was forty-nine years, with a range from thirty-one to eighty-five. This age range does not represent the age at implantation, but rather the age of the sample of women who were aware of problems tied to their implants. Based on our surveys and reviews of medical records, we know that it is not uncommon for women as young as eighteen to have implants and that many women have them during their thirties. Since national figures indicate that it takes between seven and ten years for many symptoms to appear, we are reporting here on women who have probably had their implants for some time. The median age at which women had their implants inserted was thirty-one, although the range was from eighteen to sixty-seven. The women in the current study were most likely to be between twenty-six and thirty-five years of age when they had their implants. The next largest category consisted of those between thirty-six and forty-five, these being the years described by plastic surgeons as years of "declining femininity," which make women vulnerable to cosmetic surgery.

Although other research reports that about 85 percent of the women have implants for augmentation, in our sample, slightly fewer (69 percent) but still a definite majority had implants for cosmetic purposes. Twenty-two percent had implants for reconstruction after a mastectomy for fibrocystic disease, while only 10 percent had implants after a mastectomy necessitated by cancer. This is an important point: while much of the press coverage suggests that a multitude of women who have already been devastated by breast cancer are now, as a result of the FDA restrictions, being prevented from having implants to improve their appearance, these women are clearly in the minority. Furthermore, if any women are at risk from implants, it would be these women, given that the relationship between implants and subsequent breast cancer, though not established, is suspected, especially with silicone implants.

Cosmetic surgery is often regarded as an opportunity available to upper-middle-class and upper-class women (Sullivan, 1993). The women who had breast implants were not representative of these classes in either our study or the others that have been reported (see also Kaslow and Becker, 1992). Women with breast implants are likely to be from the lower middle class, while other research suggests that women who have facelifts and other types of plastic surgery are more likely to be upper-middle or upper-class women (Pervitz, 1970). We asked women with breast implants about other surgeries they had had. While 22 percent had had no other surgery, 16 percent of the women in this group had had a hysterectomy, and 18 percent had had other cosmetic surgery, such as a facelift. They were likely to be the only member of their families who had implants (87 percent).

After a few interviews, it occurred to us that these women were, in a manner of speaking, trading on their bodies. It was essential for them to keep their bodies attractive either to get, or keep a man, or to obtain a job. In any case, economic survival, both directly and indirectly, seemed to play a role in many of the women's decisions to have breast implants. These were not wealthy women, married to doctors and lawyers, sunning in the Bahamas. Rather, they were working women, often struggling to keep a marriage or a family together, and feeling that their lives would be more livable if they looked more attractive. The single women were barely hanging onto middle-class status, or they were slowly slipping into the lower class after a divorce. Those who were married were likely to be held in the middle class by the man to whom they were married, a situation experienced by most women.

In 1995, over half of the women in our study still had implants, either silicone or saline, but increasing numbers were having them removed as their concerns about their health overshadowed their concerns about money. Most of the women (83 percent) had no idea what kind of implants they had, and almost none of them was ever informed that the implants might break or leak or cause them harm in any way. A full 95 percent were not informed of any danger from implants.

Because we have only limited information on women with breast implants, comparing those who have them for cosmetic purposes with those who have them after mastectomy, or comparing them with women who don't have implants is difficult. Even so, a profile of women who get implants is possible. Our analysis of their economic and educational characteristics, as well as our in-depth interviews with the women, indicate that they are likely to be married, nonprofessional women with more than one child, a high school degree, and jobs in the clerical or service field. Interestingly, this profile does not distinguish them from other women in this country, which indicates that they are not especially unique. They are the women next door, the women in the office, the women in line at the grocery store. It seems unnecessary to look for psychological characteristics that might lead to a desire to have implants. As we have stated, these women are responding to their economic and social reality in a culture that values women for their attractiveness.

During our interviews, over and over, we noted that the women were searching not for perfection but for improvement; not for splendid and beautiful but for "acceptable." These women were not "glamour girls" or "ladies of leisure." Rather, they were solid, traditional American women, who were happy to get the opportunity to overcome their feelings of inadequacy and inferiority about their bodies through a so-called safe, simple, and permanent surgery.

Regardless of the initial impetus for implants, the women were making an effort to conform to demands for perfection, to overcome a flaw that was either physically or emotionally debilitating, or to erase a condition that was devaluing. These reasons are not always mutually exclusive. For example, only after a divorce may some women choose to have augmentation or cosmetic surgery to correct breasts "saggy after childbirth and nursing," whereas they might not have considered it had they remained married. In their efforts to camouflage, correct, or overcome a stigmatizing condition, women often found themselves trapped in a downward spiral of pain, misdiagnosis, and disbelief. These women often did not (and did not want to) associate increasing physical problems with their implants. Once they began to tentatively link the two, however, they frequently found themselves in a battle with physicians and others but were too fatigued to fight effectively.

To recognize that a woman is attempting to overcome a flaw does not mean that she necessarily sees herself as grotesque or horrible. Rather, she may well simply think she needs improvement, fixing, or enhancement. The women in our study can be roughly divided into categories depending on the main reasons they gave for wanting implants. Although there may have been several reasons, one often appeared overriding, with the others sometimes justifying the decision. First, we will look carefully at women who had breast implants for augmentation, and then we will turn to those who had them for reconstruction.

AUGMENTATION

Women who had implants for cosmetic purposes were committed to changing themselves through surgery. Although they were more likely to have implants when going through a divorce or experiencing a strain in their marriages, not all were in this situation. Seven basic reasons were involved in getting breast implants for augmentation purposes: to erase a perceived or real deformity; to turn back the clock; to improve their self-image; simply to have bigger breasts; to make a practical, economic choice; to get a "new lease on life"; or to keep their marriage intact.

Erasing Deformity

These women viewed themselves as suffering a deformity, such as inverted nipples or breasts with misplaced nipples. Some women whose only problem was the size of their breasts seemed to fit into this category because they saw their size as a deformity, a stigmatizing condition that they had to hide from others.

Some women were so ashamed of the size or shape of their breasts that they dramatically shaped their feelings about themselves and their interactions with others. Karen had implants to overcome what she saw as a stigmatizing condition—what she referred to as a "pigeon breast" by which she meant that her breast bone protruded. She is a slim and lovely person, married with a five-year-old child, and working on a graduate degree in geography. She spoke hesitantly, expressing sadness and loss, as well as fear of the future. Her body had bothered her a great deal ever since she first became aware of sex and her sexuality. She researched the risks of implants as much as she felt she could and compared them with other solutions for her deformity. The doctor explained the procedure to her, assuring her that implants were perfectly safe and would never break. The only complication was that they might harden, in which case, he said "We'll take care of that with a capsulotomy— hitting them to break up the scar tissue." Could they break? Only if she were "in a terrible accident and were struck in the chest with a steering wheel in which case you would probably die anyway."

Betty, an older woman, artist, and television producer, rested after her nurse helped with her morning routine of bathing and dressing. She spoke softly about her first love and how she lost him because her embarrassment over her small breasts prevented her from having an intimate relationship with him. This woman, sitting in her small apartment, still reflective of the graceful lifestyle she once enjoyed, remembered this loss with a sharp pain. She had implants when her co-worker's intern husband told her that he needed someone on whom to practice his surgery skills. She "knew" it was safe and easy, and she was thrilled with the possibility of finally having "life-size breasts." Given her current painful life, she regrets that she didn't appreciate simply having a healthy body.

Another woman, middle-aged, formerly athletic and energetic, now preparing for her fifth surgery to remove silicone and repair her esophagus, bitterly recalled her father's reference to her breasts as being "as flat as Kansas." Such comments, among several other references to her small breasts, resulted in her never letting her husband see her naked. She eagerly sought a surgeon for breast implants as soon as she could afford the surgery.

Still other women spoke of breasts that were misshapen, too long, too flaccid, too stretched, nipples inverted or turned out or otherwise flawed which could be corrected through implants. These women were all trying to overcome a damaged sense of self which was intimately tied to their breasts and a feeling of flawed femininity.

Turning Back the Clock

The women in this category had at one time been satisfied with their breasts, but, after nursing children or growing older, evaluated their breasts as sagging, droopy, or not as full and attractive as they had once been. These women wanted to recapture the shape they had when they were younger.

Lacey is a beauty consultant, fifty-five years old, but looks like a woman in her early forties. Twelve years ago, when she worked for a plastic surgeon, he offered free implants to his staff in lieu of a raise. She thought it was a marvelous idea, especially since her breasts were softer and looser than they had been. Although she was leery of silicone, he reassured her that the implants were made of saline, and "since your body also consists of saline, they can cause absolutely no damage, even if they break." (Instead they were silicone implants, which she discovered only when she had them removed.) She eagerly had the implants and had absolutely no difficulty until recently, when she began experiencing a rapid deterioration of her health. Now she would choose her aging body over the body she wanted surgically changed if only she could turn back the clock.

Nancy had implants at twenty-five. She had breast-fed both of her babies and "had no breasts left," even though she had been a "C" cup before nursing. She was going through a divorce at the time, but like many women, she said that she did it for herself: "I just felt self-conscious about my breasts." The doctor told her that nursing had broken down the breast tissue and suggested an implant. After years of illness following the implants, she had them removed along with a substantial amount of tissue. She is very sick, very disoriented, and hates how her body looks—"I have to look at this every day."

Mary had her implants in 1980 after reading a good deal about them and finding a doctor she liked. He showed her different sizes and promised she would "go to the grave" with them. She had always had small breasts, and after nursing, she developed stretch marks on them. Sixteen years later, she had the implants removed because she was so sick. She now "only has a nipple." She loved the way she looked and felt with implants and would have them again if they were safe.

Renee had implants when she was twenty-eight, after her son was born. She said that she "just hated" her breasts—they hung from her "like sagging skin with a nipple on the end." She couldn't stand herself with her clothes off. There was one style of padded bra that she liked, and when she could no longer get it, she went with a friend to her plastic surgeon and made an appointment to have implants. After having the implants out, she now, once again, has "sagging skin with a nipple on the end." The only difference is that now she is sick.

We met Nadine at a local restaurant in an older part of town. She is petite, thirty-four, attractive. She was eager to tell her story and brought a folder of her medical bills and other records. Like so many women we interviewed, she had implants about a year after giving birth to her daughter, when she was in her early twenties. She was also going through a divorce but insisted that she just had implants to feel better about her breasts. Her doctor translated her efforts to retrieve a lost body, a lost self, into postpartum ptosis. She had implants for fifteen years and had them removed when her joint pain, fatigue, and memory loss were devastating her life.

Love My Breasts, Love Me

These women defined their decision to have implants solely or almost solely in terms of their poor self-image and their desire to improve their self-esteem. They merged their value as women with their breasts, and were convinced that they would be happier, more attractive, more valued, and hence more valuable if they had larger breasts. Some women in this category had almost always blamed their small breasts for their poor self-esteem, while others felt abandoned and useless after a divorce and wanted implants to boost their feelings about themselves.

Sitting in a coffee shop with a frightened twenty-one-year-old woman who had implants at age eighteen, I empathized with her reasons for having them and with her crippling fear of having them out. She had chosen to have implants in hopes that they would make her beautiful, lovable, and happy, that she could become a model, and the plastic surgeon she consulted reinforced that belief. He understood that she "wanted to be more of a woman," and diagnosed her with "micromastia." This young woman, with not even a high school education, no family support, and only dreams of a happy future saw changing her body as a way to gain value. The reaction of men to her new shape initially gave her a sense of value. Even as she began to recognize the emptiness of the words of love and desire, they warmed her in a way she desperately longed for. Her sense of self was so fragile, so dependent on others' evaluations, that even when she became sick, she was afraid that if she had the implants out she would be discarded by people who were now giving her attention. This young woman never became a model for she was simply one more ordinary looking girl struck by the dream of instant fame. Unfortunately, as a result of silicone, she began to suffer from fatigue, fever, body aches, nausea, headaches, and other symptoms that would plague her days and disturb her nights. Finally overcoming her fear of being left with hanging skin and a scarred chest, she had the implants removed.

Another young woman, Dawn, had always hated her flat chest. Her mother and sisters, shorter and rounder, had large breasts, and this lithe, sunny young woman always felt masculine and awkward around them. When she saw a television interview with transsexual men and saw their large and real-looking breasts, she immediately made a decision to have implants if she could possibly afford them. Within two weeks she had an appointment with a plastic surgeon, and she soon sported "C" cups, feeling "whole" for the first time in her life. Her friendly nature blossomed with her new confidence, and her life moved happily forward, only to be devastated two years later when she developed painful arms and knees, silicone nodules in her neck, headaches, overwhelming fatigue, and dizziness. Her implants had ruptured, and her chest wall had to be scraped to remove the sticky silicone that had adhered to her breast tissue.

Janie had breast implants so that she would finally feel better about herself. After years of humiliation about her breast size (once an employer had stuffed her bra with a sanitary napkin to improve her cleavage), she had implants after she and her new husband moved to a state where she knew no one and where he began to spend hours after work with friends from the office. She felt lost and unattractive, and decided, with encouragement from her husband, to have implants. He went with her to the first meeting with the plastic surgeon to select the cup size. She, like so many other women, initially loved her new look, feeling more feminine, sexier, more desirable. She finally "felt like a woman." She too became sick after a few years. Janie resisted the association between implants and illness for several more years, until her health was so bad that she had them removed. She is still sick, and although she has been active in support groups and lobbying efforts, she recently abandoned almost any activity that required her to leave her house.

Dana had grown up with parents who drank heavily, and as a young woman she had very negative feelings about herself, especially about her small breasts which she said were "an issue" for her throughout high school. She married a man for whom she "was never enough, not good enough, not pretty enough," an evaluation consistent with her own. Because her small breasts had always bothered her, during one of her visits to the gynecologist she asked about hormones as a way to increase her breast size. He had a pair of implants in his desk, showed them to her, gave her literature to read, and told her they were perfectly safe and would last a lifetime, much easier and cleaner than hormones or other alternatives. That night, she and her husband performed a little ceremony—they burned her padded bras in the fireplace. She was twenty-five and knew she was doing the right thing. Everything went well for the first five years, except her marriage. Her husband began to refer to her breasts as her "going away presents" since her sense of self improved so dramatically after her implants that she wanted a different life. She is representative of the majority of women who have implants—to improve their confidence, their self-esteem, to feel more attractive and more womanly.

Bigger Is Definitely Better

Some women just wanted bigger breasts. These women didn't want implants to overcome a deficit or self-esteem problems. Rather, they insisted they just thought it would be wonderful to have big, full breasts. They thought they would be more attractive, happier, and sexier, and they simply wanted them. To paraphrase some of the women, "I wanted to be the best I could be," and "since I knew I could improve my looks, I just wanted to."

Marilyn was, at mid-life, living for fast cars, good food, and handsome men. She made a lot of money on a property transaction and thought the world was her oyster. She had three facelifts before she thought about having her breasts done. She felt like she "was on a roll" financially, she had a new marriage, and she wanted the best of everything, including breasts. When we interviewed her twenty-five years after her implants, she was using a walker, weighed about ninety pounds, and was dying of esophageal immotility—she couldn't swallow because of tracheal scleroderma.

May was one of several women we interviewed who received breast implants as a job benefit. She worked as a receptionist for a plastic surgeon, and instead of paying for their insurance, he "gave all the girls implants." She didn't give much more thought to having implants than she did to changing her hair color. She thought she looked great; she loved being bigger and would have kept them if she had not become ill.

Better Living Through Bigger Breasts

These women saw themselves as making a practical, economic choice. Advancing in their career of dancing, entertaining, or serving was impossible without bigger breasts. Women who were dependent on tips saw big breasts as an economic asset. Women who danced in topless bars or strip clubs or who were showgirls in Las Vegas knew that their employability was tied to their breast size, and so they made rational decisions to have implants.

Nora is a soft-spoken woman with creamy skin and short, blonde hair. She looks like she just walked off the tennis court. She was a thirty-year-old cocktail waitress, earning pretty good money, including tips, at a casino. She never had really disliked her body or thought about implants, but two of her co-workers got them, and showed her the astonishing results. She thought they looked wonderful. Her friends loved having them and said it was a relatively easy, painless procedure, "worth every penny," which in 1975 was $1,500. After talking it over with her husband, who was favorable, she decided to get them "to improve my appearance, to feel better, being a cocktail waitress." She realistically appraised the cost-benefit ratio of having implants and decided that having bigger breasts would prove an economic advantage. Nevertheless, she never felt completely comfortable with her decision to change her body. She felt plastic and embarrassed. Her children didn't know she had implants until twenty years later when she had them out because she had become so sick.

We spoke with two dancers who had implants for similar reasons; implants would improve their chances to compete for the show parts and dance positions they wanted as they got older. Both Raeanne and Sue had implants to look sexier and better in their costumes. They spoke of their decision in matter of fact terms—it was simple economics.

Supporting the Sagging Self

These women had not always felt bad about their bodies, but as they aged, especially after a divorce, they felt old and discarded and saw implants as a way to regenerate their enthusiasm for life. When their marriages became difficult, their husbands had affairs or they went through a divorce, they thought bigger breasts would make them feel younger and more desirable. The ending of their marriages, especially facing economic problems and caring for children, left them feeling depressed and degraded, and to redeem their value, they decided to change their bodies. Some of these women wanted to remarry, and they clearly saw having desirable bodies as an essential first step. Without attractive bodies they would not be able to compete in the mating game. Others, while not so focused on remarriage, felt that larger breasts would make them feel better about themselves, helping them overcome the depression and sense of worthlessness they felt after a difficult marriage and divorce.

Marie's story is illustrative. We met her at her house in a quiet little neighborhood by a small lake, surrounded by trees. She was petite and sparkling, wearing a tight jade tank top and matching shorts; she had shoulder-length black hair, loosely curled. She had been a cocktail waitress for years; earlier she went to college for a couple of years and did secretarial work. She was twenty-seven when she got her implants, because she wanted "a better body image" after a second divorce. She thought her breasts were too small, and she had stretch marks after nursing her three children. After she saw "before and after" pictures in a magazine and read how pleased women were with implants, she discussed the matter with other women at work. Finally, she found a doctor she trusted and had them put in. She had never really thought about having implants until the divorce. Then she felt so "at loose ends," so "adrift," that she felt that having bigger breasts would help her "tie her life together" again.

Brenda, at forty-two, is happily married to her second husband and has two grown children. She had implants almost a decade ago, when her first marriage was faltering badly. She saw breast implants as a "way to make me feel better about myself. I was so young, so miserable, flat-chested and in a horrible marriage." Indeed, she felt good enough about herself after the implants to leave the marriage, move to a bigger city, and start over. For her, the implants were a vehicle to an improved self-image and a better life. After a divorce, some women feel so bad about themselves and their future that they decide to get "better breasts" to make them feel valued again.

The women who saw implants as a way of ending their depression and getting into the marriage market were aware that their bodies could be either an economic asset or a liability. This was especially true of those women who were entering the competitive dating arena and had children to support and wanted to be as attractive as possible. Implants were a way to get over feeling dispirited and "over the hill" and to compete more equally with "a lot of younger girls out there who were looking for the same thing."

I'm Begging You, I'll Do Anything, Just Don't Leave Me

These women had implants simply to keep a man or to preserve their marriage, either to prevent a divorce or to keep their husbands at home. Although very few women had implants only to save their marriage, it was not uncommon for a woman to opt for implants in order to improve her marriage or because she thought her husband was wandering. Helen was an extreme example: she had implants because her husband clearly stated that he would leave her if she didn't. Janice was more typical. Her marriage was unhappy, her sense of self was flagging, and her husband was interested in someone else. For her, as for many of the women in our study, marriage was also a significant economic relationship.

Together, these personal, social, and economic factors played a role in women's decisions to have implants. As even the most hopeful reader might suspect, a marriage held together by a "D" cup could collapse fairly easily. These marriages were likely to end in divorce, often accelerated by the pain, disfigurement, and anger suffered by the women.

RECONSTRUCTION AFTER MASTECTOMY

A significant minority of the women who have implants have them after breast surgery for reconstructive purposes. The women who had their breasts removed to avoid or to remove cancer often had the surgery with more ease knowing that they would still look normal but wouldn't have cancer or the increased risk of cancer they thought accompanied fibrocystic disease. Women indicated that they thought they would be "better than new" and "would never sag" and "wouldn't ever have to worry again." Their sense was that they were really just replacing a part of their body with something better—prettier, safer, and longer-lasting.

Women who had implants after mastectomy were a vocal minority, representing only 10 to 20 percent of all women with implants. Their demands, subsidized by corporations and the ASPRS, that implants remain available are loud and forceful. They express feelings of being violated, once by their mastectomy surgery and again by the FDA's decision to limit the availability of breast implants. Their lobbying efforts on Capitol Hill and in the media have effectively kept implants available on a trial basis, with clinical followup for women who have had their breasts removed.

Audre Lorde's experience after a mastectomy illustrates the cultural demand that women at least have breasts. She wrote that, after her mastectomy, if she did not wear a prosthesis, nurses and doctors would respond to her as if she were breaking the rules, refusing to be a woman, denying her femininity and their right to see her as a normal female (1980). Prostheses are made to look and feel "like real breasts," and women are expected to replace the missing body part rather than to compel the viewer to know they are without a breast. It is both polite and essential to the smooth flow of interaction. Basically, breasts are "givens"—they simply are a part of us, they define femininity, and they are "taken for granted" as a component of womanhood.

There were two categories of reconstructive surgery: That following mastectomies for fibrocystic disease and that following mastectomies for breast cancer. While in both cases the woman had a mastectomy, the way the surgery was explained and the way she incorporated the implants into her life were somewhat different.

Avoiding Cancer, Avoiding Stigma

In the 1970s, women who had painful, lumpy breasts and who had a family history of breast cancer were encouraged to have a subcutaneous mastectomy and implants. These two things went hand in hand—the mastectomy was presented as getting rid of a potential evil and replacing it with something better than new.

The majority of the women who had mastectomies had been persuaded to have their breast tissue removed as a preventive measure. These women, thousands in this country alone, were diagnosed with fibrocystic breast disease based on the fibrous tissue in their breasts. Women in this category often had mothers and aunts with either fibrous

breasts or breast cancer. The general medical wisdom was that such fi-
broid tumors, coupled with a history of cancer in the family, were a
precursor to the development of cancer. Today, the medical profession
has largely abandoned the label or diagnosis of fibrocystic disease, recognizing that fibrous breasts are commonplace among women of childbearing age; fully half of the female population have this condition.
Because of the availability of implants and their heavy marketing to surgeons, doctors probably saw a "win-win" situation when they encountered a woman with fibrous growths in her breasts. They could remove
the risky tumors by way of a subcutaneous mastectomy, insert breast
implants, resulting in a far lower possibility of cancer and breasts that
were larger, fuller, safe, and designed to accompany a woman to her
grave—and they could benefit financially at the same time.

An older woman, retired from her job as an accountant, illustrated the
feelings of most women facing mastectomy after a diagnosis of fibrocystic disease. Her feelings about the surgery were very positive—she
would be protected from cancer, of which she was very fearful. After the
surgery, she thought the implants were beautiful and made her feel wonderful about her body . . . she felt "better than new."

Another woman had painful, lumpy breasts and was very worried
about getting breast cancer. She couldn't tell if the lumps she was feeling
were a danger sign or just benign lumps. Having a mastectomy seemed
not only reasonable, but also a way to alleviate her worry about herself.

Regaining the Self

These women were presented with implants as the last stage of surgery to remove breast cancer. They were offered an opportunity to avoid
the stigmatizing scarring and flatness that they would otherwise experience. Women who have breast cancer are often grateful for the availability of implants, although certainly not all women choose them after
mastectomy. With the hope of a normal, relatively unscarred body, the
women we interviewed faced cancer surgery more easily. The problem
came later, after women got their implants and not only had to cope
with healing from a major surgery, but also to endure breasts that were
hard, painful, leaking, or ruptured.

Anna, a young housewife in North Dakota, had nursed her mother
through her illness and eventual death from breast cancer. That experience convinced her that she would do anything it took to survive, and
if that involved a radical mastectomy, she would simply be reasonable
about it. When her doctor told her that she could have implants to replace her breasts, she was initially hesitant. She thought it wouldn't

bother her too much not to have breasts. She had always had small breasts, and her husband didn't seem to be especially drawn to her breasts. But because of her youth and her attractiveness and "because of their safety," the doctor pressed her to consider implants. Indeed, she was perfectly satisfied with her body after the surgery. She quite liked her new look, and she kept it for years, having the implants removed only after years of illness.

Jocelyn was only thirty-four when she was diagnosed with breast cancer. She had recently remarried and had a seven-year-old daughter. Breast cancer terrified her; the visual image of having her breasts removed, having stitches in her chest, and the actual surgery frightened her almost more than dying of cancer. When her surgeon assured her that she would look "like new" with her high, firm breasts (she could even choose the size), she underwent the mastectomy with high hopes and even a little enthusiasm.

These categories reflect some of the different reasons for having implants and capture the diversity among the women. For the most part, the women went into the surgery with great hopes, expecting only the best. As a result, they were loath to acknowledge that their subsequent problems might be tied to their implants. However, they did experience a wide range of problems of both a localized and systemic nature. While not all women experienced the same problems, the overlap and repetition was astounding, as was the response these women received from their plastic surgeons.

7

The Aftermath and the Stigma Path

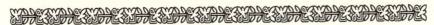

First, she is evaluated according to an idealized criterion she usually falls short of and is ultimately destined to transgress, and second, her natural, bare and uncontrolled body is unacceptable.

Tseëlon 1995, p. 89

THE AFTERMATH

So, women reconstruct their bodies and, they hope, their lives. Their problems with self-esteem and relationships, their worries about the inadequacies of their bodies, and hence, of themselves, are redefined as medical problems that can be solved with enough money and a little courage. After a woman has implants, the next chapter of the story begins to unfold, a chapter in which she may become sick, her implants may harden or move, silicone may travel throughout her system, and she becomes fatigued, with aches and pains and a flu-like illness. This is the part of the story she didn't anticipate. This is the beginning of her awareness that although her breasts may not have been perfect, they were better than what she now faces. She also learns that while the plastic surgeon was happy to redefine her small breasts as a disease, he is not so eager to view the complaints she presents as a result of the cure he has offered. The aches, fatigue, pain, and other problems she now encounters are likely to be defined as psychological in origin or a result of menopause and its attendant complications. She finds herself pursuing medical care in a climate of disbelief, one in which physicians, family and friends are likely to question her assessment that her illness is caused by her silicone implants. Her reality is seldom shared by others and even she often wonders whether she is not simply depressed, or suffering symptoms of menopause . . . or maybe losing her mind.

WHAT HAPPENED?

Research on postsurgery satisfaction suggests that even when the results were not as expected, women were quite likely to be satisfied with their implants (Fee-Fulkerson et al., 1996; Kaslow and Becker, 1992). Some women thought their implants did not look perfect, but liked the way they looked in clothes so much better that it didn't matter. Others, even if the doctors thought they could look better, were well-satisfied with the results. For some of the women, problems began immediately, problems such as infections, hardening of the implants, improper healing, or uneven and misshapen implants. For many of the women, however, it would be months, often years before they experienced any problems. And it would often take even longer for them to associate their pain with the implants, finally doing so in a "climate of disbelief." They frequently encountered doctors, strengthened by pressure from the AMA and the ASPRS, and eventually by studies conducted at prestigious institutions, who didn't believe them. Had these women had one consistent symptom or if their symptoms had formed a perfectly predictable constellation, they might have been believed. If they had not been between the ages 40 and 50 when they began associating their symptoms with their implants—a time when women were likely to be defined as premenopausal, menopausal, postmenopausal, or simply aging—they might have been believed. In fact, if they hadn't been women it is quite possible that they would have been believed, especially if we infer from studies illustrating physicians' differential reaction to men and women who have headaches, backaches, and chest pain (Khan, 1990; Wallen, 1979).

PHYSICAL SYMPTOMS

What were the symptoms these women experienced and when did they occur? Among the women who responded to our questionnaire, a large number reported numerous physical problems. In almost two-thirds of the cases (70 percent) the problems resulted from rupture in which the silicone had migrated to the women's collarbone, neck, arms and other parts of their bodies.

Almost all of the women reported general aches and pains, breast and chest pain, fatigue, memory loss, numbness, and Sjögren's syndrome. The vast majority also reported severe headaches, body rashes and abdominal discomfort, and almost half reported hair loss and scleroderma.

These are the common physical complaints of women with breast implants as reported in numerous studies. Women who wrote the FDA about problems with breast implants (271 letters, January 1, 1992–July

31, 1992) complained of the following local reactions: breast pain (40 percent), rupture (31 percent), and fibrous capsule (29 percent). The most common systemic problems were joint pain (39 percent), fatigue (35 percent), and muscle pain (13 percent). The women also reported, though less frequently, fever, rash, dry eyes, and hair loss (McCarthy et al., 1993: 112). An earlier study from Australia (Varga et al., 1989) reported autoimmune connective tissue disease after mammoplasty, and numerous reports from the United States suggested a relationship between connective tissue problems, such as scleroderma (a very serious connective tissue disease), rheumatic diseases, and weakness, fatigue, muscle pain, and joint pain and silicone breast implants (Bridges and Vasey, 1993; Merkatz et al., 1993; Simon, 1995).

Connective tissue disease associated with silicone gel implants was first reported in 1982 by Van Nunen and colleagues. In 1988, an article in the *Journal of the American Medical Association* reported scleroderma in women with breast implants (Speira, 1988). Other studies followed, reporting patients with silicone gel breast implants and scleroderma, systemic lupus erythematosus, undifferentiated connective tissue disease, Sjögren's syndrome, rheumatoid arthritis, and other diseases (Bridges and Vasey, 1993). In 1992, studies investigating the relationship between breast implants and connective tissue disease and arthritis were reported at the American College of Rheumatology annual meeting. These studies of over 750 patients investigated the relationship between breast implants and connective tissue disease and arthritis. Most patients had nonspecific symptoms of myalgia, arthralgia, and fatigue, although more than 130 cases of connective tissue disease were reported. The most common were rheumatoid factor negative, inflammatory arthritis, and scleroderma (Bridges and Vasey, 1993). As Speira reported in 1988, these women were not sick before their implants other than having the usual number of colds, flus, and surgeries. Subsequent to the implants, they began suffering significant problems, although often these were not initially associated with the implants.

Women, whether having implants for augmentation or for reconstruction, had a difficult time accepting the possibility that the "solution" to their felt problem was indeed a new and potentially devastating problem itself. Many women reported that they initially linked their symptoms with recovery from surgery in general, with overwork or stress, or with lupus or arthritis or some other disease. Some women, even when they strongly suspected the association between their illness and their implants, refused to have them taken out, fearing not only the surgery but also the maiming and disfigurement they expected to accompany surgery. Actually, the degree of disfigurement is very dependent on such factors as whether the woman had a mastectomy, whether her implants ruptured, and if so how long before she had them removed, and the care and precision of her physician.

Some women, desperately ill, so dread the consequences of removal—the hanging skin, the sagging, concave chest, the ugliness—that they refuse to have the implants removed. Some women are very pleasantly surprised at how good their breasts look when they have the implants out. Simply having the implants removed will not guarantee a return to health. Many women who have had their implants removed still suffer many of the problems they had, because while the implant may be gone, the silicone that leaked or ruptured into their body is still there, impossible to fully remove.

LATENCY PERIOD

Many of the women we talked with (18 percent) began having problems immediately after the implants were inserted. Sometimes the wound would not heal, and often the implants caused extreme pain, they hardened, or moved to other places in the chest cavity. During the first year, another 16 percent began to have significant problems such as hardening of the breast or so-called capsular contracture and chest and breast pain. Hardening of the breast and loss of nipple sensation are the only two problems of which women are usually informed.

Whereas about one-third of the women began to suffer immediately or during the first year, by the end of the fifth year almost 70 percent of the women had one or more of the common symptoms. Other studies (Brautbar et al., 1995; Simon, 1995) generally report that symptoms are not likely to appear until eight to ten years after the implant, but the women who responded to our questions reported their appearance earlier. This may be because our sample consisted of women who were sicker than other women, or who were not representative because they were more involved in the medical and legal fight over implants than other women with implants. It may also be, however, that many women experience symptoms long before they associate them with their implants.

Among the women in our sample, only 16 percent had their first problems ten years or more after they had implants. Fully 84 percent had experienced problems before that time. Among the women we talked with, almost 40 percent had their implants replaced at least once due to hardening, rupture, or some other problem. Vasey and Feldstein (1993) conclude that all implants will eventually rupture or bleed and that at some point all women will have to have them replaced or removed.

Many who suffered the consequences of rupture were not aware of the rupture until the implants were removed. The silicone had been largely captured by the scar capsule that formed around the implant.

The women we interviewed were consistently poorly informed about their implants. Most of the women (84 percent) had no idea what kind of implants they had, either the first or subsequent sets. Some were told nothing, while others were given incorrect information, such as that they had saline implants when in fact they had silicone. Most of the women gave the distinction between silicone and saline implants little thought and simply relied on their doctor's choice. Furthermore, the women, almost without exception, were told that the implants were absolutely safe; they would not break, rupture, or bleed.

These women had to deal with much the same problem faced by women who are raped: disbelief on the part of those to whom they report their problem, in this case, the doctors. Many doctors suspect that the million or so women with implants are reporting symptoms they have heard about through the media, much as rape victims are accused of being talked into the idea that they were raped, or making it up the morning after to protect their reputations or sense of self (Roiphe, 1993). Some even believe they are experiencing some sort of hysteria.

What do the women say about what happens to them? Over eighty women in our study described how they connected their illnesses to their implants. Their experience is typified by that of Charlotte Mahlum, plaintiff in a successful suit against Dow Chemical Company for approximately $10.2 million in punitive damages and $4 million in costs. During the trial in 1995, she looked wan and weak, but, like many of the women, she didn't look deathly ill. Her relatively calm demeanor hid her unremitting and increasingly disturbing illnesses. She matter of factly related her history as follows.

Charlotte had a double mastectomy, recommended by her physician because of fibrocystic breasts and a family history of breast cancer. He insisted that she have implants because of her age (35), because he had "seen marriages destroyed by mastectomies," and because they were safe and would last a lifetime. "He made me look in the mirror after the mastectomy; he said that a lot of women go off their rocker and need treatment after removal." Because she had a mastectomy, expanders filled with saline were first placed in her chest, made larger progressively until they would accommodate an implant. When she was first implanted, she developed a severe infection and had to spend weeks in bed. Her twelve-year-old daughter brought her food and water and changed the dressings on her wound. Immediately after implants were placed in her body, they became very hard, like baseballs; they were also cold and sometimes moved spasmodically in her chest. Her breasts would change color, red to pink to blue-white, and move around in her chest. She felt like she was "carrying three bricks on [her] chest." Charlotte lived with this pain, increasing sleeplessness, and headaches for almost ten years, sometimes feeling well enough to work, at other times being incapacitated.

Although she was accustomed to hard work, having grown up in a big family in a farming area and working as a waitress five days a week, her fatigue and pain required her to reduce her time to four workdays, then three, and soon, because she couldn't trust her legs to hold her or her arms to carry the heavy platters, she had to quit. No one except her daughter and her husband knew she had implants. She lived in a rural area and knew no one either in her community or in her family who had ever had implants. She was afraid to mention it for fear that she would be seen as vain or self-important. After almost ten years of pain and fatigue, her daughter, now grown and working for an attorney in a larger city, told her mother about the hundreds of cases she had seen which sounded just like hers—the hair loss, memory loss, fatigue, sleeplessness, pain, itching, and crawling sensations. She tried to get her mother to go to a doctor, but Charlotte refused. The symptoms were too elusive, no one would believe her, and she was embarrassed to talk about either her body or herself.

She finally agreed to talk to an attorney, Geoffrey White, whose background in cases involving the sedative L-Tryptophan and autoimmune responses had led him into the area of breast implants. He referred her to a doctor who would be sensitive to her symptoms. The doctor examined her and found that her implants were ruptured and would have to be removed. Charlotte couldn't face another surgery. The first was so painful, the recovery so slow, and the appearance of her chest so unpleasant without breasts, and she was in so much pain, that she dreaded another intervention. But the doctor insisted that the implants come out. Her husband, assuring her that he didn't love her for her breasts, also pushed her to have them out. The implants had been ruptured for a long time, several years, but because of the scar tissue capsule that had formed around them, she was unaware of the rupture. The doctor had to scrape silicone from her ribs and chest wall but was unable to remove it from the area under her arms and around her ribs. Vacuuming and scraping the thick, sticky substance that had adhered to her tissue and bone resulted in a concave chest, vertically and horizontally scarred—a devastating outcome.

Charlotte noticed a slight improvement in her health after the implants were removed, but the relief was short-lived and soon the original symptoms returned, stronger than ever. To this day, she experiences a consistent crawling sensation "like they took a pine box and put you in it so you can't move and fill it full of night crawlers so they crawl all over your body—you feel like you could just rip off your skin to stop the itching and crawling." Charlotte loses control of her bowels, she has no libido, and she can barely tolerate her husband's touch. She walks with a cane because she loses her balance even walking across the room, she has numbness in her arms and legs, and she suffers severe headaches and searing pain in her chest. She anticipates a shortened life, one spent in pain. She has stayed alive for her granddaughter, an elfin girl who looks like her grandmother and who is her namesake. She plans to give her body to science to demonstrate the impact of silicone.

Who believed her? Some doctors, some experts, and a jury. Dow Chemical's effort was to prove, first, that silicone was inert, or if not, that it wasn't dangerous if it leaked or spilled, and to demonstrate, second, that even if it was dangerous and if they didn't test it adequately, they still weren't responsible because they only manufactured the silicone gel, not the implant itself. The jury was unconvinced. It found Dow Chemical responsible for Charlotte's illness, for fraudulent concealment, for negligent undertaking to aid and abet Dow Corning, and for fraudulent misrepresentation. The jury, appalled by Dow Chemical's callous disregard for Charlotte and hundreds of thousands of other women, awarded approximately $4 million in compensatory damages and $10.2 million in punitive damages against Dow Chemical. At present, Dow Chemical is appealing this case to the Nevada Supreme Court. Charlotte Mahlum, now divorced, lives perilously close to death.

Another woman, also part of the public record even though her case against 3M/McGhan settled during the trial, was far more obviously ill than Charlotte. Mildred Merlin was dying; no one on either side of the case debated that. What they did debate was the cause, with the defense claiming the problem to be related to smoking and other lifestyle factors and emotional trauma, and her attorneys claiming that it was due to silicone leakage and her body's autoimmune response. During the trial, she weighed less than eighty pounds, and she could barely breathe or talk. She was alive, she said, to have her day in court, to tell her story. I worked with her before the trial to help shore her up to face the kind of questioning she might experience and the stress she would surely encounter. Mildred had smoked, she had lived a full, nontraditional and colorful life, and the implants were just one reflection of that life. Yet, for her, the issue wasn't about her morality or her citizenship, but about the fact that she was dying from what she was convinced was silicone poisoning. The defense's reliance on the Harvard and Mayo studies was anticipated, and while powerful, was not so persuasive that it could overcome the obvious illness of this very frail woman. The case settled during the trial for an undisclosed amount.

Marilyn Halverson is yet another woman dying of silicone; specifically, she is dying as a result of esophageal immotility, according to her medical records. We met her during Charlotte Mahlum's trial. She had traveled from Seattle to give her support with a nurse/companion who accompanied her everywhere. She was wraithlike, almost bald and very unsteady. Her story was an interesting one. Coming up from poverty, she was a self-made woman who enjoyed her notoriety as "the wild Norwegian," an entrepreneur and contractor. She had implants in 1969, at 31, while in a new marriage. Her left breast had always been slightly smaller, and when she began to develop cysts in her breasts, she was easily convinced that implants were the solution. Implants would allow her to have beautiful breasts and still nurse her babies. She would "have beautiful breasts when she was 100," she was told. She thought it was a splendid idea. She loved dancing, driving her white Corvette, living on the wild side. Implants seemed a perfect complement to her exciting life. Today, in her long white-blond wig and her dramatic clothes, she is a ghostly reflection of the flamboyant woman she was. She wants her granddaughter to remember her as a flashy, loving woman, not as this person "drooling in a wheelchair." She endures every day with what resembles a severe flu—headache, body ache, nausea, sleeplessness, crawling skin, dry, painful eyes. She has a scleroderma-like disease of the esophagus that is destroying its elasticity. She suffers night sweats, swollen lymph nodes, intermittent blindness in one eye, brain lesions, and inflammation of the pericardium. She knows she is dying. Despite all these symptoms, she has no hope of a settlement, for there are no punitive damages in the state of Washington.

And what of young Mara who had implants at eighteen to make her feel like a worthwhile woman? Soon after having the implants, she complained of a great deal of pain in her breasts but no sensation in the rest of her chest and no sensitivity in her nipples at all. When she returned to her plastic surgeon, alarmed after several weeks of such pain, he accused her of lying because she hadn't called earlier to mention these problems. This very timid young woman had been too worried, too full of self-blame to go to him, because he told her the only problem she could have would be hardening that would result if she didn't massage her breasts enough. When she finally went to see him because she could no longer tolerate the hardness and pain in her breasts, he performed a closed capsulotomy squeezing the breasts and hitting them to break the tissue apart.

Her worries continued. When she lay down, a large lump protruded from the side of one breast. Her surgeon said there was nothing wrong. Her husband finally took her to the hospital, and an ultrasound revealed a fold in the implant. While the physician at the hospital could not tell whether or not her implants had ruptured, her plastic surgeon discouraged her from following up on the matter "because they're just trying to make big money on you." After that, she didn't go back to that doctor. Her symptoms have worsened during the subsequent two years; she is extremely fatigued, feels weak, and sleeps a great deal. She is dizzy and feels "blurry"; her mind wanders and she cannot concentrate. Her speech is slurred, and she suffers severe depression. She, like at least half of the women in this study, is taking an antidepressant. When she lies down, the lump still protrudes from the side of one breast. She has sought the advice of two other doctors about having the implants removed. One doctor insisted that there was no evidence that implants caused any problem; the other, more sympathetic, ordered blood tests and encouraged her to have the implants taken out.

One of the women we talked with knows she should have her implants out but is paralyzed with fear and depression. She says: "The process is real hard. You have to always see a new person, show them your breasts, they want to touch them, you have to reveal yourself. I hate to show them. I feel like an old woman, I want to be a better wife and mother, but I'm too tired." This young woman knows she will have them removed, but struggles more painfully with that decision than she ever did with the decision to have implants in the first place.

Lyn had implants after twenty years of marriage mainly because her husband wanted her to have a better body. Her implants were larger than she wanted, but both her husband and the doctor decided that her frame could accommodate them. She never liked the implants and was embarrassed by her body. She avoided friends, feeling maimed and humiliated with these large breasts. She experienced trouble and pain from the time she first received them. She tore one of the implants when lifting something heavy soon after the surgery. She subsequently experienced severe pain in that side and arm, even if she tried to lift anything "as light as a bowl of cereal." She has had three surgeries on her left breast—twice she has had the implants replaced. For the first year or so after the initial implants, she said she had to be "popped" every month or so. Lyn is agitated and cringes as she talks about the terrible pain and horrible sounds that accompanied these closed capsulotomies. After injecting her with Valium, her doctor would exert enough force to the breast to break apart the hardened capsule. She says she could hear a tearing, then a hot rushing from the breast, as if blood or liquid were oozing from them, "like you've been cut badly." He sometimes had to do the procedure five or more times to break the hardness. She cried from the pain and the humiliation.

Lyn was so degraded by this experience that she told no one, not even her mother, she had implants. Her doctor insisted that the hardening was the result of her failure to massage her implants. She was so tired of the closed capsulotomies and her shame and humiliation that she finally decided to have the implants removed. Her doctor, saying there was absolutely no evidence of any connection between implants and illness, refused to perform the surgery, saying she would hate the way she looked. He, like so many, insisted that "when you die, you'll be the only corpse with big, beautiful breasts." (Given this common refrain, one begins to suspect that big breasts are far more important than the woman's life.) Lyn insisted that the implant had to come out, despite arguments that they were perfectly safe. She began to refuse blame for the hardening, insisting that this was happening *to* her, not *because of* her. Finally, while also insisting that she was "blowing this all out of proportion," another surgeon agreed to remove them for $6,000, money she didn't have.

From 1986 on, she suffered severe chest pain, pain so severe that at one point she had a heart attack and was not aware of it, so accustomed had she become to the incapacitating chest pain. Her hands ached and were tingly and numb; her hair, once thick and healthy, became thin and brittle. Her fatigue was overwhelming, but no doctor associated these symptoms with her implants. Rather, they attributed them to her hysterectomy. Finally, three years later, a doctor suggested she have the implants taken out, but she still had insufficient money. It was not until she found a doctor who would take payments that she finally had them removed. She discovered that her right breast had ruptured so severely and had been ruptured for such a long time that it was necessary to do a great deal of scraping and "cleanup work" to get the silicone out of her chest cavity.

Today, Lyn is severely scarred, her arms have knots of silicone in them, and she cannot lift anything heavier than a lipstick. Her fatigue and aches are sometimes immobilizing. She has absolutely no hope that she will improve in the future.

Dawn was the first person I interviewed. Her doctor had told her she had "Snoopy complex," his attempt at a humorous description of long, droopy breasts. She was thrilled to have implants at twenty-six and felt good about her appearance. A couple of years later, she was in a serious automobile accident, requiring plastic surgery on her face. Because she thought she had saline implants, she was not concerned about them, thinking they would have deflated if they had ruptured. Soon, her breasts hardened into two tight balls, and she began to feel worse. She had not told her husband that she had implants, and she didn't want him to touch her breasts. She began to tire easily, to have arthritis- and rheumatism-like symptoms, a low red blood count, neurological symptoms, and some symptoms consistent with Epstein-Barr syndrome. She felt a lump in her right breast, and although ultrasound revealed no problem, a biopsy showed that not only did she have silicone implants rather than saline as she believed, but also that her implants had ruptured. She went back to the surgeon who had placed the implants in her chest, and he refused to take them out, saying that she would be totally flat and would look "grotesque." Dawn had a chronic infection, and she was sure it was due to the implants. Still, she feared being misshapen and maimed. Since there was no agreement that the implants posed any problem, she simply waited, with ruptured implants, not sure what to do. She finally had them removed by a surgeon who had done her facial repair several years earlier. The doctor subsequently did a mammoplasty that involved lifting the breast tissue so there would be no droop. The surgery was far less intrusive than the first, which had involved deep incisions to create a space for the implants. She feels good for the first time in years.

Dana said the surgery itself was "a piece of cake." She loved her new breasts, at 34B not large by anyone's standards, but perfectly satisfactory for her. The first five years seemed fine, even though she had to have one implant replaced. Then, when she was around thirty, she began to have minor but increasing problems, chronic low grade fevers, bladder infections, and pelvic inflammatory disease. She eventually had a hysterectomy. She seemed to "catch everything that came along"; she had no resistance and low energy. She saw several doctors, who asked if she had any problem with her implants. They looked fine, she liked them, and they didn't hurt. Her reply was "No problem." She was loath to admit any problem—she loved how she looked, and felt, and she wanted to keep them. She couldn't imagine going back to her flat chest.

Finally, after months of extreme fatigue and hardening breasts, she did decide to have the implants removed. One ruptured during the surgery, and because the other implant had ruptured and calcified earlier, a great deal of her chest tissue had to be scraped out. "I slept in a chair for months, my body was so sore, I was so worn out. It felt like electric shocks were running up and down my body for weeks after the surgery." Fearful of being disfigured, she had saline implants as soon as she could, but she continues to feel sick.

Depression and cognitive difficulties are especially problematic for

Dana; she feels like she is in a stupor. At forty-four she will receive a medical retirement from her demanding and responsible job—the first person in her state to receive a medical retirement based on atypical connective tissue disorder. But she will experience a significant financial loss, to say nothing of her personal loss, and she now fears that her cognitive abilities will diminish to the point that she won't be able to hold down even a menial job.

These women with breast implants consistently face the discrepancy between the treatment they received when they considered implants, whether for augmentation or after mastectomy, and the treatment they were accorded when they became sick. Generally, when a woman seeks consultation for breast augmentation, the atmosphere is one of professional interaction between patient and doctor, strengthened by a medical definition of the problem and a medical solution. When the woman seeks to have the implants removed (often by the same doctor who placed them), she is treated as though she is doing something wrong. She is considered an alarmist, held responsible for her own problems, and is not treated as a legitimate patient seeking a medical solution to a medical problem.

Danielle's experience is a good example of the shabby treatment such women get from doctors. When she finally convinced her surgeon to remove the implants, she was rushed in and out of his office. The implication was that she was slovenly or careless in insisting on the extreme and defeminizing procedure of having the implants out. Her experience with the doctor convinced her that he saw her decision as an attack on him and his judgment, and she was treated as an outcast rather than as a patient.

Danielle's experience was not unique. As previously stated, many doctors refused to remove these women's implants, and the women believed they were defined as blameworthy and inconsiderate for wanting them removed. In our interviews, the women posited that the doctors had such a large stake in the implants being safe that when they were presented with the possibility that the devices were damaging, they turned against the women who brought them the information. This occurred when women had capsular contractions or other pain associated with the implants, when they reported illnesses they thought might be related to the implants, and when they wanted the implants removed. In contrast, they had been treated as legitimate, reasonable, and right-thinking women when they decided to have them inserted in the first place.

These experiences illustrate that women with breast implants face not only medical and legal but social problems as well. They usually have implants to overcome some sense of inadequacy, they subsequently suffer significant medical problems, and finally they face difficult and tiring legal battles. The painful emotional experiences these women continue to have can be understood within a framework of their efforts to overcome or avoid social stigma and the successes and failures in those efforts.

THE STIGMA PATH

Women face a powerful paradox—the demands to be beautiful and young mask the insidious evaluation of them as essentially ugly. The requirement to remain attractive is built on an assessment of woman as morally and physically unworthy, needing camouflage and deception to appear even acceptable. This fundamental ugliness can only be conquered by daily attention to the details of their bodies, vigilant oversight of weight, skin, hair, feet, all imprisoning the mind through the constant attention required to control the body. To fail in this control, to improperly bind or support or cover or reveal, implies moral failure, and slovenliness of the person and makes the self unacceptable. While the media engender a deep and constant insecurity about their physical appearance in all but the most secure women, they simultaneously recognize they are dependent on positive evaluations of their appearance (Chapkis, 1986:40; Tseëlon, 1995:78). Therefore, women are sometimes willing to go to dangerous lengths to improve their appearance and battle aging through endless diets and unsafe, unnecessary surgeries. The interplay between the images presented through the media and the expectations of others, including doctors, parents, and lovers, is crucial in our self-assessment. As Schur points out, appearance norms are a "central element in the objectification and devaluation of females," and concern about meeting these norms pervades women's lives (1984:66). Restrictive and unattainable appearance norms draw women to a mirror in which they are endlessly flawed. Women hold this looking-glass to themselves, viewing themselves as objects to be scrutinized and evaluated, leading to a daily life for women that can be accurately described as a "dizzying series of mirrored images of bodily stigma, of failure, interpreted as moral failure" (Schur in Valentine, 1994:119).

This failure can be overcome, or at least atoned for, through a willingness to alter the body, to perfect oneself as a "sight," a perfection that requires the internalization of the male gaze, leading the woman to evaluate herself the way a man would (Spitzack, 1990:53; Valentine, 1994:120). Her reflection is less directly related to any objective recording of her visual reality, her thighs, her waist, her mouth, her breasts, than to all of the depictions of the perfect female form. This form represents values that are translated through the media to the "significant others," to use Mead's terminology, with whom we interact, and who reinforce these male values, having unwittingly incorporated them into their world-view. As Goffman (1976) points out, beauty for women is an identity claim that is taken on faith only as long as it can be sustained. Sustaining it is women's consuming work because the claim is to a conditionally spoiled identity. Only through hard work can the woman avoid being shown as ugly, destroying her claim, spoiling her identity. The success of her presentation of self to others determines her evaluation of self-worth.

For women, having no breasts, or "inadequate" breasts, is a stigma, and many women obtain implants in order to overcome that stigma. Goffman (1963) defines as stigma all the deformities and character blemishes that interrupt the ongoing flow of social activity. The stigma may be immediately visible to others, as in the case of blindness or perhaps cerebral palsy, or it may be hidden, such as is the case with epilepsy or diabetes. Such stigma either discredit the individual outright or have the potential of doing so. Discrediting stigma are those that immediately devalue the individual in interaction; they are visible and immediately disruptive of the interaction. Discreditable stigma are those that would devalue the person if others were to know. In either case, the individual must manage the stigma and find a way to hide or incorporate the offending characteristic in order to allow social interaction to proceed with as little disruption as possible. One might even emphasize a discreditable or discrediting characteristic in order to have it dealt with by the other immediately, hoping that it will then fade into the background.

The deformity or shameful secret influences not only the interactions in which the stigmatized engage, but also their decisions about whether or not to engage in interactions, with whom, and under which circumstances. The self-knowledge is so intimately tied to evaluations of the self that even though the stigma is invisible, it is powerfully shaping. Women who wish to conceal the size of their breasts or other such problems have easy access to clothing and devices such as padded bras, loose clothing, and prostheses which create the illusion of normality. But the women themselves know that they are presenting a false image of self. Their own information about their bodies would devalue them if others were to know. They must therefore manage encounters with others (i.e., manage the stigma) by carefully evaluating the "who, when, and where" of disclosure. They run risks, as do all people with discreditable characteristics (e.g., those with herpes, epilepsy, or diabetes), of offending or losing other people if they time their disclosure incorrectly or if they misjudge the reaction of the recipient of the news. They must therefore be concerned with the stigmatizing condition and with its impact on the other as well as on the self. When women have implants for cosmetic reasons they experience yet another stigma—that of having breast implants. So while they may gain large or perfectly shaped breasts, they also are often perceived as having done something irrevocable and abnormal to their bodies. The stigma path continues when women have their implants removed, because now their condition is often worse than the initial condition they were attempting to correct.

Many of the women we interviewed felt they suffered a stigma and readily embraced the possibility of erasing it through breast implants. As Lenore stated, "My breasts were always small, I was almost flat. I couldn't let anyone, even my husband see me without clothes. I just didn't feel like a woman." Suzanne's father told her, "I thought you were a boy," and his nicknames of "brother" and "buster" humiliated and shamed her. She knew breast implants would make her feel whole. Karla's reasons were also representative: "I just always felt awkward and awful about myself. I was badly burned when I was a little girl . . . on my back, but I thought if I looked more feminine, that wouldn't matter as much."

Other women avoid potentially stigmatizing events through implantation. They were so frightened of getting cancer, of losing their breasts, that they eagerly agreed to have mastectomies to remove calcifications or fibrocystic growths. Irene said:

It was no big deal. I went in by myself and took a cab home. I just had these lumps, calcifications, and the doctor thought I should have my breasts off so I didn't get cancer—no trouble, nothing to worry about. He also said he'd plump them up . . . they were shrunken down after nursing, but nothing to worry about.

Deena had fibrocystic disease at the age of twenty-seven, and the doctor told her they "had to come off."

I said "no way." My mom had one [mastectomy] and my dad divorced her. He said he didn't want to be married to "half a woman." But I had to take care of my mother and watch while breast cancer killed her. I changed the dressings; it smelled awful. I just couldn't face that.

A minority of the women underwent mastectomies after being diagnosed with breast cancer. They avoided stigma by having implants as the last step in their surgery, and even though they were not quite as "good as new," these women compensated for the loss they experienced to save their lives. Heather told us: "I had to have a hysterectomy at twenty-six. Then I got breast cancer and had a mastectomy a few years later. The implants were supposed to just replace what I lost." Similarly, Joanne reports: "I was so relieved when I was told I could have breast implants after my cancer surgery. My mother had cancer too and a radical mastectomy and I saw what it looked like. My doctor told me if I was his wife he'd give me implants."

Still others felt stigmatized, not so much because of the size of their breasts, but because they had been divorced or deserted and their imperfect bodies represented their devalued selves. These women seemed to have a very poor sense of self, to view themselves as inadequate and unlovable, suffering not only a physical but a moral stigma as well. Goffman writes about physical stigma as well as flaws of character. These women viewed themselves as flawed humans, and steeped in American culture, they viewed their bodies as representations of themselves. As Jane illustrates: "I was so depressed after my divorce, even though he was an alcoholic and I'm better off without him. I just felt awful, so old and useless and angry. I felt like breast implants would make me feel better about myself." Ellen reports much the same feeling: "I just never felt good about myself. I wanted implants to build me up, to let me know I was a woman and could mean something to somebody."

Most women with breast implants were initially pleased with their implants, enthusiastic and happy with the way they looked. Many of them clearly felt that they had overcome the stigma of small or misshapen breasts. We frequently heard women say that they felt like "real women" for the first time, that they were elated with their bodies. Their self-esteem skyrocketed, and they felt desirable, attractive, feminine. Such feelings about the self sometimes led to significant changes in their lives. Some left a bad marriage; others felt confident dating, or better about their appearance or their jobs. It was not until they became ill, or when the implants ruptured or moved, or became misshapen that they experienced dissatisfaction. Even then, some of the women were afraid to have them removed, or decided that the risk of further illness was worth the benefit of having large breasts. One woman I interviewed, Alice, had to have four surgeries to remove the silicone from her chest after her implants ruptured. This woman, married to a successful professional, busy with her children and volunteer activities, was nevertheless eager to have implants again. Her physician warned her about the possible problems with implants and cautioned her against them. She promised to wait until her health improved to have them, but she was insistent on having them, especially because of the way her chest looked after the surgeries to remove the implants. She said she "just didn't feel like a woman with such a flat chest."

STIGMA ADVOCATES

Even though there are overwhelming cultural messages about breasts and femininity, these messages are filtered through social interactions, either being weakened or magnified by the very particular and unique nature of these interactions. Definitions of the self and evaluations of self-worth are embedded in groups and relationships. People with whom we are closely involved are influential in our decision-making process because of the strong messages about general culture and the more specific expectations they carry. Women do not evaluate breasts or bodies in a social vacuum, nor is the decision to have implants made in isolation. They are aided in this process by what might be called stigma advocates—those people, either professionals, family, friends, or media figures, who are involved, first, in defining a problem, and second, in defining it as one that can be solved through breast implant surgery. These stigma advocates build on an already established milieu that encourages women to view themselves as imperfect and potentially stigmatized and that establishes the physical self as a reflection of moral worth.

In consumer society, as Valentine points out, the media act as a very powerful "other," the "mediated generalized other" in the development of individual identity (Meyrowitz, 1985). They instruct us about "average" and "normal," often setting impossible standards and doing so through "homogenized images of perfect and perfectible bodies" (Edgley and Brissett, 1990:271).

Because the appearance standards for women are so narrow and at the same time so unwavering, ignoring the diversity of the female self and body, women find that they never measure up. They are never enough, yet they remain a spectacle, being seen from everywhere. Valentine (1994) suggests that the imperative for bodily perfection comes less from others and more from a mediated relationship with the image of women on television and in the other media. Indeed, the media are powerful conveyers of standards that may change but that nevertheless demand perfection. These standards are reinforced, built upon, and made salient in our everyday interactions. Others serve as a conduit for the transmission of cultural values, reinforcing those displayed in the media.

Parents and other significant family members are important translators of media images and interpreters of the cultural world. Women may have been encouraged, purposely or unwittingly, by a spouse or father to see their breasts as inadequate, to see themselves as less than feminine. Male evaluation seems especially important in the development of an identity problem, a stigmatized condition. Yet it is often other women, sisters or friends, who help the woman make the decision to have implants once she entertains this possibility. The off-hand remarks, the subtle messages received by these significant others, meld with the media images of big-breasted women as valuable and attractive to encourage reconstruction and perfection.

Husbands sometimes acted as stigma advocates for the women we interviewed, encouraging them to get implants, even saying they would leave them if they refused. We may remember Jay, Helen's husband, who stated that if she had implants he would "have something to stay home for." Other women reported that their husbands had helped choose the size or had pushed for implants either directly or through criticisms of their bodies. However, the women in our study who were currently married were almost without exception married to very loving, supportive, patient men. Marv Mahlum accompanied Charlotte to every doctor's appointment if he could get off work; he also did the housework, helped her get dressed, and cleaned up after she lost bowel or bladder control. Bill held Dee's hand during our interview, telling her, "I don't love you for your breasts, I love you for your soul." Often the men accompanied their wives to our interviews, helping them fill in the information they had forgotten, adding to their accounts of the experiences with doctors.

Other stigma advocates are the plastic surgeons who build on the cultural demands for acceptable bodies for women and who represent the legitimate medical system's response to a woman's problem. These physicians help a woman mold her dissatisfaction into a medical ailment. They can transform a droopy breast into a medical disease, postpartum atrophy, and small breasts into micromastia, thereby legitimizing a medical intervention. Whether women have implants for cosmetic purposes to enhance their breasts or have reconstruction to re-create their breasts after surgery, they build on an obligation to meet cultural ideals of femininity.

The legitimation and decision-making power of doctors is apparent both during the period when a woman is deciding to have implants and when she is deciding whether or not to have them out. If she is having them for cosmetic reasons, she, of course, sees a plastic surgeon who often encourages her to have the implants. The surgeon is in the position to medicalize her deviance, small breasts, and he has the full support of the manufacturing industry as well as his professional associations. Plastic surgeons validate her desire for large breasts by offering her a medical label for her dissatisfaction with her breasts, such as postpartum atrophy, or involutional ptosis. They also encourage her by simply agreeing that her breasts are too small or too long or too narrow or too misshapen.

Professional associations to which the doctor belongs provide the background and justification for the medicalization of women who want implants, and reinforce the woman's view of herself as having discrediting stigma. Plastic surgeons support breast augmentation, indicating that the purpose of all aesthetic surgery is "to improve the quality of life of the patient through enhancement of his or her self-image" (Biggs et al., 1982: 449). However, because cosmetic surgery (in this instance breast implants) involves altering healthy anatomy that falls within the normal range of variation, the questionable legitimacy of such procedures demands a redefinition of such variations as deformities, as deviation or stigma eliminated by body manipulation. As with other types of plastic surgery, physicians are united in their view that women's concerns for their appearance are essential to their nature as women. Women are required to "achieve gender," to act and dress and be consistent with gendered expectations related to their sex. And for women, this achievement is never an accomplishment; it is always a process, and increasingly with age, a losing proposition. As Dull and West (1991) report, because plastic surgeons see women as accountable to particular sex categories, they also see women as "objectively needing repair" (64).

ILLNESS AND RESTIGMATIZING

In the case of breast implants, a significant lobbying effort, directed at both the FDA and doctors and women, has been launched to convince everyone that not only are implants safe, but small breasts are in fact a *disease* requiring medical intervention. Recall that in 1992, when the FDA was investigating the safety and efficacy of implants, the American Society of Plastic and Reconstructive Surgeons claimed that "There is a common misconception that the enlargement of the female breast is not necessary for the maintenance of health or treatment of disease . . . these deformities (small breasts) are really a disease, and . . . the enlargement of the underdeveloped female breast is therefore, often very necessary" (Zones, 1992:236).

This "disease" received the name "hypomastia" or "micromastia" and evidently is relatively common. This conceptual medicalization—redefining a normal phenomenon as a disease rather than a normal variation—provides the background for the institutional medicalization of which Conrad and Schneider (1992) speak. This phase of medicalization allows individual medical practitioners to validate the woman's problem by applying a new definition of the situation—that of a disease—and then to intervene medically to correct that disease. Physicians, ordained with a great deal of legitimate authority, can actively transform normal body variations into "objectively problematic conditions" (Dull and West, 1991). This expansion of medical authority has transformed the aesthetic realm into a terrain ready to be mined by medical practitioners.

The medical context and potential for stigma is somewhat different for the process of reconstruction after mastectomy. Although the structural aspects of the medical sector remain important, it no longer becomes necessary to provide an account for the surgical intervention because breast implants are seen as part of a natural and anticipated progression in the healing process. The intervention is viewed as legitimately correcting the previous "surgical mutilation," getting the woman "back to normal." In this case, the reconstruction prevents the stigmatizing condition of having no breasts and normalizes the woman who would otherwise be discreditable. With breasts, she can remain a "real woman."

Small breasts, as we have seen, have been transformed by the ASPRS from a normal variation in breast size into a disease. But, simultaneously, most physicians and all of the implant manufacturers, as well as the ASPRS, deny the physical and medical consequences of silicone gel leakage or implant rupture. Those most eager to claim small breasts as a disease are also most adamant in their denial that their treatment could have caused any problems for the patients. In each case, the construction of the situation may be seen as tied to financial and status benefits for the medical establishment.

Over four hundred thousand women in the United States now claim that they are sick as a result of silicone breast implants, but they make this claim in a climate that denies their illness. The women we interviewed had an extremely difficult time receiving any legitimation of their illness. So unsupported were their claims of illness that they often thought they might be becoming mentally ill. Even they began to doubt their judgment, to question the validity of their pains and other symptoms. Women who have had implants and who have become sick have come full circle to another form of stigma. Many of the women we interviewed, who had placed a great deal of emphasis on their bodies, and who felt that their identity, their femininity, was linked to their breasts, have now had their implants removed. In the process, they have lost not only tissue, muscle, skin, and their health, but also a major piece of their identity. Darla's response to her body is illustrative:

> I am so ashamed. . . . I never even look at myself in the mirror. I won't let my husband see me, or touch me. I live in my own hell. I live in fear he will leave me because I'm so sick. I try to tell myself I can fight this, but I hate my life, and I know if I get worse, I'll kill myself.

Charlotte felt sick, weak, and dispirited: "When my implants ruptured, I hurt so bad I didn't care if I lived or died. One day, I was driving and just thought of running into a semi. I just didn't think I could stand going through it anymore."

One woman we interviewed said, "Feel me, I'm concave." Several other women now have "nothing but scars." These are women who have had silicone leakage, whose implants have ruptured, who had to have the implant and capsule scraped and cut from the muscle. These women, sometimes after years of trying to convince numerous doctors that they were sick, finally decided on their own, not with the collaboration and support of physicians, that the implants needed to come out. They have sometimes felt better after removal, but often, especially if the implants had been in for fifteen to twenty years, their symptoms of fatigue, aches, connective tissue disease, skin discoloration, hair loss, headaches, and memory loss have not improved. These women now not only have no breasts, but they are sick, sometimes disabled, and usually unable to support themselves.

These women are confronting difficult questions of identity as discredited or discreditable persons. First, they chose surgery as a means of avoiding or overcoming stigma but as a result of this choice, they may now suffer even greater stigma as well as experience emotional discrediting. Their claims to feminine identity are in jeopardy. If, as Tseëlon (1995) suggests, women are required to work to maintain their gender, to avoid being discredited, and to maintain their claim to femininity, women who have had their implants removed face an absolutely herculean identity battle.

Women have responded in a number of ways to the discrediting information they possess. Some women feel disfigured: one woman said she would not go to her mailbox without her prosthesis, and she would no longer let her husband caress her during lovemaking. She feels her relationship is ruined, and her fatigue makes her unable to reclaim it. Another woman we interviewed, Charlotte, said that she no longer feels like a woman—she is "cut to the bone." These women express anger at themselves for their "stupidity," for not knowing the implants were dangerous, and anger at their doctors for implanting them in the first place. Further anger is reserved for the doctors who now deny that their sickness is related to implants. For the women who feel disfigured, shame and sadness accompany the anger. These women are not likely to speak at support group meetings or to publicly disclose their disfigurement.

Other women, perhaps surprisingly, some who placed great emphasis on their appearance, have dealt with the disfigurement and the scarring by publicly announcing the damage they have experienced. They have become actively involved in lobbying efforts, have taken leadership roles in support groups, or have acted as support persons for others at work or in the community. They have funneled some of their anger and pain into efforts to help others in similar situations, and they have begun to achieve a certain status and significant identity as spokespersons and organizers. They have basically dealt with the stigma of disfigurement by disclosure and declaration, asserting their validity.

Many other women waver. They reveal selectively, telling a daughter, for example, but not a lover, about the implants and their impact. Some women will participate actively in a support group meeting but protect their identity at work. Two of the women we interviewed were very careful that no one saw us interview them or overheard our conversation. The preservation of the sense of self in their social world demanded that they be perceived as "whole, real women."

In all of these cases, women must decide how to construct a presentation of self in an environment of disbelief. Very few of the women we interviewed had doctors who supported their assertion that their illnesses were related to their implants. Often friends and family were initially sympathetic toward them, but having read the newspaper reports and seen television programs about the safety of implants, had a difficult time remaining supportive, especially since the symptoms women had were obscure, sometimes fleeting, and followed no regular pattern. These very characteristics also made the women vulnerable to self-doubt.

PREVENTING STIGMA

A number of the women reported that their physicians were not willing to remove the silicone implants unless they replaced them with saline implants. Especially for younger women, or women who had no "significant other," physicians insisted on replacing the implants to protect the women from disfigurement. The women reported their physicians saying such things as, "You will hate yourself unless you have replacements," "Your husband won't want to look at you if you don't replace them," "You're too young to look like that," or "Men lose it when they see their wives like that." Such demands by physicians were also powerful denials of the link between implants and disease. So, even when women could come to terms with not having breasts and were willing to have the implants removed in order to get well, even when concern for their physical well-being far outweighed concerns with their appearance, their physicians insisted that "women's concerns with their appearance are essential to their nature as women" (Dull and West, 1991: 64). Physicians demanded that women conform to their notions of the physically acceptable female, despite potentially devastating consequences. Physicians' insistence that these women fit their construction of femininity overwhelmed their concern for the woman's health.

The understanding of women's experiences with their decisions about breast implants, and the consequences of these decisions, can be elucidated by understanding them as attempts to avoid or overcome stigma, to conform to gender demands. Women who get breast implants are conforming to the American ideal, whether they are replacing or enhancing their breasts. Ironically, this very effort results in physical and medical damage to the extent that these women are often mutilated and deformed. The stigma they then have to manage, while still related to their breasts, is of a different nature and requires complex management techniques. Women who have breast implants illuminate cultural demands to achieve gendered ideals, and they suffer the severe and sometimes debilitating consequences of such efforts.

8

Medical Records: Negotiated Reality

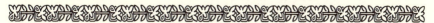

> ... illness is a social construction based on human judgments of some
> condition in the world. In some fashion, illness, like beauty (and like
> deviance) is in the eye of the beholder.
>
> Conrad and Schneider, 1992

This is the "information age." From infancy to death our "vital statistics"
as well as seemingly endless not-so-vital pieces of information about us
are recorded. These records follow us from place to place, job to job,
hospital to hospital, therapist to therapist, even marriage to marriage.
Some of us are outraged at the lack of privacy accompanying this age,
the transformation of humans into numbers, the reliance on charts and
social security numbers and data rather than on *us*, the people about
whom the records are made. Others appreciate the convenience and ef-
ficiency provided by the reliance on records. But no matter how one feels
about it, it is clear that records are a substantial part of most of our
interactions with any bureaucracy, whether we're registering our children in preschool or licensing our automobiles or trying to balance our
checkbooks. We begin to anticipate our records proceeding or accompanying us, and we accommodate ourselves to the demands of recordkeeping.

"Just a minute, I'll pull up your chart," or "What is your social security
number, I'll find your file," or "let me get your records," or "bring her
inoculation records with you" become background expectations as we
interact with any bureaucracy. Clearly, this makes a certain amount of
sense; there is no need to re-create one's medical history each time one

sees a physician. An advisor must rely on a student's records to assess the student's progress, and an insurance company needs the client's records to accurately evaluate one's coverage. It is an undeniable reality that records also become more than just documentation of activities or behaviors or statements. All records are made within a context, a social, interactional, and political context, and the record ultimately consists of the meanings established in this context. Rather than being a neutral transfer of information from source to recorder, the record is instead a construction created by the interaction of two or more people in a social context. If we are talking about an academic setting, for example, grades reflect a number of things: the performance of the student, which in itself is based on expectations and assumptions, the expectations of the teacher, which are influenced by the student's sex, race and class, the characteristics of the school, the characteristics of other students, the parent's involvement, and often such elusive factors as the teacher's acceptance of or appreciation of the student.

In a similar fashion, medical records are a reflection of a dynamic process that occurs between doctor and patient in a social context and against a backdrop of expectations both people bring to the examining room. The doctor's training, cultural background, gender and gender expectations, as well as the patient's expectations, physical signs or symptoms, ability to articulate, and class, race, and sex of both physician and patient shape the interaction. The cultural setting of a series of interactions in which the doctor is often of superior status, often male, in control of the interaction and in which the patient is usually of lesser status, female (in the case of breast implants) and dependent on the doctor, and in which there may be great social distance between doctor and patient, with varying abilities to communicate and empathize with one another is also determining.

This doctor-patient interaction takes place within a larger context in which professional socialization incorporates stereotypes about women and health, and in which the structure of the medical profession infantilizes patients and creates dependencies on physicians for service and help. This interaction is embedded in cultural stereotypes, myths, and expectations about health, sickness, gender, race, and class. From this, a record is constructed that is extremely complex and initially tentative, but that eventually becomes a solid construction of reality. The record begins to stand for us, to stand in place of us, to replace us, and to precede us in the interaction. The record is relied on not as a construction occurring in the complex interactional setting described above, but rather as a statement of fact, a reflection of reality, a truth. Herein lies the problem, a problem that becomes a primary determinant in the breast implant controversy. We need to deconstruct the relationship between doctor and patient, to tease apart the interlocking pieces, and to reconstruct it as a separate reality that may have only a tangential, and a not entirely predictable relationship to the pieces of which it is formed.

THE RECORD

Medical records are political constructions, reflective of activities engaged in by people with different amounts of power and different access to information, who jockey for the ascendancy of a particular definition of reality. The record is an accomplishment of at least two people engaged in a very complex process. It is necessarily so, reflective of a process in which a patient seeks a doctor's care because the patient first defines something as wrong and second defines that "something" as having its roots in some problem of the body that can best be understood and addressed by a person trained in medicine. Symptoms and diagnoses are negotiated by both participants with varying degrees of clarity and understanding.

Even if there is a clear understanding, the information presented is not left "raw" but is funnelled or sifted into categories by the physician, who draws on the background assumptions that are brought to the interaction. Assuming that there is clear communication and that the patient presents signs that are consistent with symptoms of particular diagnoses reasonably available to the physician, all of this complexity must be recorded, often by a hurried physician, in a short-hand, efficient manner. There is indeed no assurance that every sign presented, every symptom understood, every potential diagnosis is recorded. The record is not even a summary; it is in fact a selected presentation of interpretations based on a diagnostic interaction. It is a construction, truly a reconstruction of reality.

Let us turn to the patient's role in the construction of the record. Actually, the process begins when a person seeking to become a patient presents what she sees as her problems to a doctor or, more accurately, a whole series of doctors, who are then responsible for diagnosis and record-making within the context of an interaction. The women bring to their consultations with physicians cultural lessons in hierarchy and power relationships which influence the interaction. They bring cultural recipes about gender interactions and expectations, which also have a shaping influence on the interaction. In addition, they bring their undifferentiated physical symptoms, as well as their fears. After these initial visits, as they go from doctor to doctor, they begin to incorporate anger, self-doubt and self-blame.

THE PATIENT

In this political environment, the woman brings knowledge of her dependence on the medical profession as a whole and on this particular practitioner. This situation is reinforced in a number of ways, including terms of address, characteristics of the setting, waiting to be seen, determining the parameters of the discussion, and the like. Status cues abound: she is referred to by her first name, while the doctor uses a title; she waits for the doctor rather than the other way around; she enters the physician's environment which is established for his rather than her convenience and ease; and the physician determines the direction of the conversation, indicating not only the relative value of the information she is providing, but also deciding when the discussion begins and is completed. This interaction is situated within her previous experiences with the medical profession and her awareness of the respect and admiration due those in that profession in our culture. Her efforts to communicate her signs of illness are enmeshed in her desire to be helped. This desire may be tainted by her fear that she will not be believed or taken seriously, a fear that may result from previous encounters with other medical professionals. Although the woman may represent a "clean slate" to a particular physician, she is not a clean slate to herself. Rather, she is a compilation of previous presentations and reactions, diagnoses and treatments, hopes and disappointments.

Women with breast implants who are sick are women in search of an answer. Often, their efforts not only do not provide an answer, but they also result in a sense of failure as well as anger and self-doubt. The women begin to question themselves after receiving different and conflicting diagnoses, or hearing again and again that there is nothing wrong with them. At some point in the process, both the doctor and the woman may begin to doubt the reality of the woman's many signs and symptoms. Both may entertain the possibility that she is malingering or "just going through the change" or is "simply depressed." The process is an enormously difficult one for the women, one in which they often receive no satisfactory explanation for their fatigue, pain, sleeplessness, and other complaints. They may never convince their doctor that their implants are related to their symptoms, even if the doctor agrees to remove them. The steady efforts of manufacturers to convince doctors of their safety erodes what little credibility the women have. In addition to generating self-doubt, these many trips to many different specialists can work against the women later in court where they may be used to portray them as "hypochondriacs" based on the frequency with which they have sought medical care.

These women often move from doctor to doctor seeking help from different ones at different times for different symptoms, and they seldom assess the interactions as very helpful or informative. This frequent changing of doctors lends an air of incredulity to the complaints presented by these women, who are already, from their physicians' perspectives, likely to be rather tenuously connected to the truth. Yet there are good reasons for the numerous visits to different segments of the medical establishment, for the symptoms resulting from silicone leakage are complex, subtle, and wide ranging (McCarthy, 1993). Not all physicians, by any means, believe that silicone leakage causes problems, nor are they familiar with the types of symptoms associated with silicone. The women are often dissatisfied with the diagnostic abilities or attitude of the physicians whose treatment they seek. Of course, not all physicians are reluctant to see a silicone-disease relationship, and some are actively supportive of the women. Certainly, some physicians have been cooperative enough to evaluate the woman's symptoms and place her on the disease grid which was established in the multidistrict, global settlement. But they do not have to believe there is a relationship between implants and illness in order to do so.

Rene, who had implants at thirty-two, after she and her husband of fifteen years were divorced, reflects the reactions of many of the women to their medical consultation: "It's hard to make doctors understand that you could hurt as bad as you do—if the x-rays and regular tests look 'OK,' they assume you don't know what you're talking about. No one hears you."

Irene put her doctor's response very succinctly, saying: "He just didn't think implants could cause that kind of chest pain." Janice, a forty-three-year-old married accountant who has had implants for ten years, said of her first visit to a doctor for the pain she was experiencing: "He gave me a chart of the body and asked me to mark the places where it hurt. When I marked the whole body, he just didn't believe me. He said I couldn't know what pain was if I could mark so many places."

As time went on and women sought medical help from different specialists, they began to experience a great deal of self-doubt because their own experiences were so seldom validated by the doctors. Diane, who has silicone lumps under her arms and up the side of her chest, fibromyalgia, dry eyes, dry mouth, backaches, and headaches, reflects this experience: "People just cannot know what it is like, it is so hard to describe the pain I feel. You can go from doctor to doctor and they just don't think anything serious is wrong with you. It makes you feel like an idiot."

Sometimes their doctors simply dismiss them as hypochondriacal, as was true for Jenny. Her doctor said she should see a psychiatrist because "you need a better understanding of your body and what pain really is." Lenore reports a similar experience: "I hate going to the doctor. You go in with a complaint and come out feeling like you're out of your gourd."

These experiences lead to frustration in women's attempts to have their problems diagnosed, and women are likely to become increasingly angry, fearful, and ashamed as they continue their search for an answer and for treatment.

INTERACTION AND NEGOTIATION

Both women and physicians bring to the diagnostic interaction a set of "taken-for-granteds" about the world, a meaning system that is the cultural setting for the evaluation of signs, diagnoses, and treatments. It is within this climate that women attempt to gain treatment and cure for the disease they experience. It is within this climate, not a neutral, sterile, medical environment, but one charged with political posturing and the specter of litigation, that the diagnosis and treatment take place. This is the environment in which the medical record is generated, and its impact on the record is crucial. Yet, the medical record is presented and perceived as a neutral recording of fact, hence a representation of an objective truth. This assumption, though erroneous, continues to flourish among laypersons as well as in the courtroom.

Medical categories and diagnoses are social through and through, having meanings generated by the activities of social groups and individuals within those groups (Foucault, 1973). Only if we see the medical record as a recording of a lifeless line in which one party presents information and another reacts can we view the record as anything other than a rich reflection of ongoing interaction, including missed cues and varying degrees of clarity and comprehension.

There is a necessary inequality in this diagnostic interaction, given the different resources that the participants bring to the setting. These resources are embedded in a system of gender relations in which women are of lower status than male physicians from whom they seek diagnosis and treatment. As Reissman (1983) says:

Women's structural subordination to men has made them particularly vulnerable to the expansion of the clinical domain. In general, male physicians treat female patients. Social relations in the doctor's office replicate patriarchal relations in the larger culture, and this all proceeds under the guise of science—in these ways, dominant social interests and patriarchal institutions are reinforced. (15)

The women and the doctors they consult attempt to construct, from the various pieces of information they have available, a diagnosis that comes closest to representing their different perceptions of the situation. Once this diagnosis is accomplished and is documented as a medical record, it is presented as representative of a truth or fact, and as such has significant consequences for the woman during litigation.

Medical records are not fact, however. Rather, they are political constructions, reflective of activities engaged in by people with different amounts of power and access to information, in which each party maneuvers for the ascendancy of a particular definition of reality.

The patient describes for the doctor a series of signs such as headaches, fatigue, aches, pains, and fever, and the doctor translates these into possible symptoms of particular problems. The doctor and the patient engage in a process of "give and take," questioning and answering, and eventually arrive at a diagnosis that is more or less reflective of the signs the patient presents. The ultimate question to be answered during this often tedious process is whether the person can legitimately become a patient. Can the person credibly occupy the sick role and benefit from its attendant qualities? Quite simply, is the person really sick? The patient has a certain range of information that can be communicated to the doctor with more or less accuracy. The effectiveness of the communication depends on the separate and interactional abilities of both parties to communicate. The physician generally searches for a sensible categorization of the signs presented by the patient, relying on their timing, severity, combination, and longevity, as well as drawing on some notion of "what's going around" or what it is likely to be, in light of the other, extramedical characteristics of the patient, such as sex, age, educational level, and race.

SUSPICION

It is on this complicated stage, complete with a particular definition of reality on the part of doctors, that the interaction between women with breast implants and doctors is played out. And this interactional setting is, of course, not static. Not only is the field of medicine changing, with new studies, theories, and discoveries being produced, but the women who come to the doctor arrive with different sets of information, given the changing landscape of knowledge about breast implants. Today, when a woman suspects her implants are causing her illness, she may present more, and different, information than she did in the past when she had no reason to suspect any connection. This has negative as well as positive consequences: she may point out signs that she otherwise wouldn't mention, such as sleeplessness or forgetfulness along with the discussion of muscle or joint pain. On the other hand, the mere fact that there is significant controversy about the impact of silicone on the immune system may lead to suspicions that the woman is exaggerating or that her symptoms reflect what she has read or heard more than what she is experiencing.

Today, as a result of the media attention given the most recent Mayo study and the Harvard Nurses Study (Gabriel et al., 1994; Sanchez-Guerrero et al., 1995) published in the *Journal of the American Medical Association*, as well as the efforts of visible media personalities, such as the media star, Dr. Dean Edell, physicians may be more suspicious of the signs presented by women than they were only a couple of years ago. For their part, the women may hesitate to present the entire range of their symptoms, knowing that the epidemiological studies that the media have so widely reported do not support their contentions that their implants are making them sick. They approach their doctors in what they know to be a "climate of disbelief," and they must direct some of their energies toward convincing themselves that their symptoms are real and important before they can effectively communicate that to their doctors. Within this climate of disbelief, the negotiation of the medical record is especially difficult. The responses that women receive from their physicians shape the subsequent steps they take in the process of seeking help for their complaints; they may return to the same doctor over and over, seek other opinions, explore other tests or nontraditional treatments, or simply give up, convinced either that there is no help for them or that they are hysterical or mad.

There is not a linear progression of the disease or of the woman's response to it which can be used to make sense of the experience. Rather, there is a scattering of signs and symptoms, seemingly unrelated in their diversity and unpredictability, which corresponds to the woman's sporadic and shotgun approach to discover the cause and appropriate treatment for her illness. The environment in which women and their doctors communicate is indeed not neutral. It is contaminated by the physicians' disbelief and doubt and by the women's fear, anger, pain, and self-doubt. The woman presents her signs within a social and historical context. The record resulting from all of this can be expected to be only partial and segmented, not consolidated as a single, clear constellation of symptoms pointing to one disease entity.

PHYSICIANS

Physicians listen to the woman through a porous screen of knowledge and potential diagnostic categories based not only on professional training but also on their immersion in the broader culture. It would be unreasonable to assume that physicians do not absorb the same culture as the rest of us do—the same language, jokes, beliefs, media images, and so on. They bring these with them, often unwittingly, into the diagnostic interaction. Furthermore, they bring the professional language and categories that they have learned in school and that have been subsequently reinforced in their formal and informal interactions with peers. Physicians are not immune to media messages, especially those that relate directly to their profession. Moreover, the professional organizations to which physicians belong funnel research findings and their interpretations to them, through articles and editorial reviews (see Angell, 1996), maintaining a constant flow of information. All of this shapes the way in which they hear and see the woman, and it forms the base on which the medical record is built. As such, it is based on a complex of signs, feelings, interpretations, assumptions, understandings and misunderstandings, and expectations.

Physicians hear the woman and evaluate her complaints heavily influenced by what Erdwin Pfuhl (1993) has termed the "theory of the office," an explanation system that is learned by the practitioner as the profession is learned. These theories allow for certain combinations of symptoms and disallow others, and they include causes and prognoses. That is, the theory of the office is an everyday, taken-for-granted language and explanation system used by professionals, in this case physicians, which reflects their training in the profession.

Physicians who specialize develop a specialized and esoteric language and explanation system. Their professional memberships, their ongoing professional training, the journals they read, and their contacts with pharmaceutical and products representatives all become part of their "state-of-the-art" knowledge of their field. This then is the information they bring into the interaction with the patient as they listen and construct a diagnosis and determine a course of treatment.

The women we interviewed reported a pattern of problems that they didn't understand and couldn't predict, and interactions with doctors that left them angry, depressed, full of self-doubt and hopelessness. The "climate of disbelief" and the doubt in which they found themselves can be separated into several categories, reflective of the range of interpretations of their experiences. That is, as the women searched for an explanation for their illness, often one that related to their silicone gel breast implants, they encountered responses that provided alternative explanations and that left them feeling confused, discounted, or incredible. Physicians were likely to respond to the symptoms and the women in several different ways and to roughly use the following categories in their assessment of the women: exaggeration, menopause, and mental illness—or sometimes, all of these.

EXAGGERATION

Many of the women reported that their doctors thought they could not have either the number, or the combination, of symptoms they reported, and such reports cast doubt on their legitimacy as reporters. Sandy, who had her implants out after almost twenty years, states that she encountered only one doctor who empathized with the degree of pain she experienced. Her chest pain has been so severe in the past that she has been hospitalized after having a heart attack, a diagnosis she doubted throughout the hospitalization. In fact, a number of women with whom we spoke reported severe chest pain and symptoms of heart attacks, which are often confusing for the physicians and for them as well.

Lonnie had implants as a newlywed after she found a lump in one breast. Her surgeon insisted that because of a significant cancer risk, she should have a mastectomy. Twenty-five tumors, all benign, were removed, and she had implants almost immediately. Ten years later she found a sizable lump under her arm and "was feeling just plain rotten, starting to lose some feeling in my left side and face, numbness and fatigue." A number of tests were run, including tests for MS and lupus, and all were negative. After three years, with the lump still there and the fatigue worsening, she insisted on removal of the implants. Doctors, who had been "pooh-poohing its importance," found that her implant had ruptured and silicone had leaked near her spine. Her implant on that side was replaced. Six months later, still feeling terrible, she insisted that both implants be removed. Her doctor, she reports, "spent about 45 minutes telling me how ugly and deformed I would be" and said he "would not be responsible for how I looked." He warned that she was overreacting and that if she got involved with the litigation over breast implants she would not be able to get a doctor to treat her.

Other women report similar reactions. Joanna had her implants taken out in another city, and when she returned home one of the wounds tore open. Her doctor, who had originally implanted her, would not resuture the wound because he didn't want to be part of any litigation. Knowing no one else, she went to the emergency room at the local hospital where her breast was stapled, as a result of which she has a significant scar.

Some doctors refuse to continue to treat a woman if she questions their diagnosis or if she provides a different interpretation of her symptoms. When Dorothy wrote her doctor a letter correcting some of his record after he had diagnosed her, he replied, telling her he would no longer treat her. Her letter was a reasonable and respectful recording of some information she thought he either needed to add to her record or use to correct some misinformation. The record was not changed.

Debra is so easily tired that she lies down on the bathroom floor after a short shower before she can gather the strength to dry herself off. When she puts on her mascara, she has to "rest between eyes" it is so difficult for her to hold her arms up. Yet, she says no doctor ever entertained the possibility that her problems could be related to her implants. They suggested she was depressed about her marriage or still suffering postpartum fatigue.

One talkative, feisty, and powerful-looking woman had implants that began bothering her within the first three years. When her implants became painful, baseball-size lumps on her chest, her plastic surgeon gave her a closed capsulotomy, which, she reports, hurt so much that she fainted. His response: "that couldn't hurt that bad; you're overreacting." These women's experiences reflect a perception that women aren't reliable or trustworthy reporters of their own experiences, and are prone to exaggeration and hyperbole, perhaps especially the type of women who would get breast implants.

CHILDBIRTH AND MENOPAUSE

Many of the women who have symptoms of silicone poisoning are in their forties and fifties, having had their implants in for a decade or so. Unfortunately, women between thirty-five and sixty-five (most of a woman's adult life) are susceptible to being defined in terms of their reproductive status—labeled either premenopausal, menopausal, or postmenopausal. These women with breast implants frequently found that their symptoms were interpreted as caused by hormonal changes, normal for women their age. This is, of course, partially understandable given some of the signs they report—night sweats, depression, forgetfulness, vague aches and pains. But it is also possible to see the willingness to categorize this diverse array of signs as menopause as a reflection of a general attitude toward women and women's health. In addition, there is the broader tendency to medicalize women, bringing natural bodily processes under the medical domain. This results in a tendency then to ignore the assault on the woman's body from a foreign substance and to normalize her pain and fatigue as part of her expected aging process, which is accompanied by the types of symptoms she presents.

A number of younger women found that they were defined as being slow to recover after childbirth, or suffering depression as a result of their new status. This tendency to implicate pregnancy or childbirth or menopause or some other problem related to woman's reproductive system simply makes the point that women are defined in terms of their bodies, and those bodies are defined as naturally problematic, if not pathological. Because women have been so heavily medicalized in this country, significant complaints are often relegated to the status of normal menopausal or postpartum adjustments. There is no need then to take women's complaints seriously, as indicative of some dire problem; they are just part of the pain naturally visited upon women.

Many of the women we interviewed felt "thrown away," abandoned by the medical profession, so great was their dissatisfaction with the results of their efforts to get adequate treatment. The astonishing fact that for decades implants were being inserted in women's bodies without even one study verifying their safety does support their feeling that their health was not a dominant concern to their doctors, the manufacturers, or for that matter, given the FDA's response, to anyone. Many of the women expressed the opinion that what happened to them would never have happened to men—neither the original problem nor the reaction to it from the physicians, the press, and the FDA. There is no good reason to disagree with them.

Sandy has severe night sweats and some disorientation. Her doctor concluded that a lot of women have these disorders because of their age. Irene's doctor, despite her numerous complaints, recorded that she is in excellent shape for a person her age. She wondered about the implications of that; should she just expect to experience pain and discomfort as normal in her forties and fifties, was he talking about "her age" as the age of menopause? If she was in this much pain now, what could she expect as normal pain when she was sixty, or seventy, if she was fortunate enough to live that long? When she questioned him, she reports that he threw the file across the table at her and walked out of the conference.

Jolene had implants after a mastectomy and now suffers extreme fatigue, joint pain, headaches, and dizziness. An MRI revealed two depressions on her brain, but her doctor has told her "not to worry . . . you are just beginning menopause and you will have that."

Many times the women themselves think their symptoms might be related to menopause, especially the "night sweats" and depression.

Sometimes these are very young women, women who have experienced these symptoms for a number of years without relating them to their implants. Because they were convinced that the implants were safe, they assumed along with their doctor that they must be experiencing some hormonal imbalance.

MENTAL ILLNESS

The third common response reflecting the climate of disbelief is to categorize the women as mentally ill or emotionally disturbed. If there is an initial assumption that women who have implants are trying to overcome some emotional insecurity, some psychic scarring, the tendency to define their symptoms as mental illness is compelling. Certainly, women are more likely to be suspected of emotional instability than are men, and they are more likely to be viewed as hysterical or untrustworthy. Therefore, it is hardly surprising that some of their physical problems are interpreted as emotional problems. Since these women are already confused by their illness, and since there is so much controversy over the relationship between implants and illness, the suggestion that they are mentally ill can be convincing, confusing, or enraging. Many women expect their doctor (or husband or friends) to think they are either hypochondriacal or attention seekers, so they are extremely defensive at the suggestion that these are psychosomatic complaints. One woman, for example, felt stripped bare by the physician, robbed of any legitimacy or power. She "was treated like a loon" and furious about it.

Irene says she sometimes feels like committing suicide, or like just sleeping forever because the pain is so severe and because she doesn't think physicians really think she could be in as much pain as she says she is. Her physical pain is matched by her emotional devastation. Being viewed as mentally unstable has had a severely deleterious effect on her.

Teresa is so ashamed of the way she looks that she won't even let her family doctor see her chest. She has chronic fatigue, rashes, and constant, intense pain. A doctor she was referred to in another state told her she had silicone poisoning. She was enormously relieved by the diagnosis, her reaction being, "You mean I'm not out of my mind?"

Lisa talks openly about killing herself "if things get worse." She tells us that her "husband was always there for me" and there was "nothing more he could have done to help her," but that she couldn't live in pain forever.

When Dee wanted her implants removed, the doctor who had been so cooperative in implanting them seemed to "treat me like I was having an abortion." He left her feeling devalued, "like a failure and dirty." He told her she would "look grotesque" and that she was "nuts to ruin a good thing."

Debra has scaly skin, extreme fatigue, disorientation, and unpredictable growths on her body. Her doctor said that anyone who had as many symptoms as she did "must have a screw loose." He suggested that her symptoms were a result of the problems she was having in her marriage.

These women are very vulnerable to the labels of mental illness that are presented to them. They are indeed depressed, often hopeless, and angry, and they have begun to doubt their own sanity because their problems are so difficult to diagnose. At the same time, they are furious with the suggestions that "it's all in your head," and they rail against the efforts to define silicone gel breast implants as safe.

RECORDS, MEDICAL EVALUATION, AND THE GLOBAL SETTLEMENT

Judge Sam Pointer demanded that attorneys for the Plaintiffs' Steering Committee and the manufacturers agree upon a "global settlement" that would provide compensation for the majority of women who were involved in litigation. These women were expected to "opt in" to the settlement, but were allowed to "opt out" at various and specific times if the terms of the settlement became unacceptable to them. If they opted out, they would then be able to take their cases to court. Given the enormity and complexity of the litigation, most attorneys encouraged all but the most obviously ill and "perfect" clients to opt in to the settlement. The women could thereby be assured of some compensation, and the attorneys would be assured of some payment for their services.

The global settlement states:

> The disease compensation program will compensate claimants who have met the diagnostic criteria for the diseases and symptom complexes listed herein. Claimants who have met the diagnostic criteria will be classified in accordance with the various Compensation Categories. (Breast Implant Litigation Settlement Agreement, 1993:1)

The committee developed a "disease grid" that categorized the symptoms experienced by the women in terms of type and severity. Women were placed on this grid after examination by a "qualified medical practitioner," who relied on seven major disease categories in the assessment. These included systemic sclerosis/scleroderma, systemic lupus erythematosus, mixed connective tissue disease, rheumatic syndrome, nonspecific autoimmune condition, as well as others (Litigation Settlement,

1993). A major component in the establishment of appropriate diagnoses, and therefore a significant component of justice as defined by this settlement, is the history contained in the women's medical records. This history, which is constructed in the records the woman brings to her evaluation, is the baseline from which the diagnostic interaction begins for placement on the disease grid, resulting in the definitional confirmation of an identity for the woman. This, along with clinical observation, blood tests, and other diagnostic tests, provides the physician with information allowing placement on the disease grid, thereby defining the degree of disability suffered by the woman and determining her compensation.

The process of reconstructing a reality from medical records takes place in court day after day during trial, and similarly results in the placement of women on the disease grid, as women are evaluated by doctors for classification into categories developed by a committee consisting primarily of attorneys. The grid categories are a tool to be used by attorneys as they represent clients, yet these categories become of paramount importance in determining how medically "disabled" a woman is. This is not only a judgment of significance for grid placement and compensation but also crucial evidence in court for determining the specifics of her illness.

RECORDS AND THEIR USE IN COURT

The use of records in court differs in some respects from their use in determining a woman's placement on the disease compensation grid. Although the financial stakes are very high, and although the record can be used to demonstrate various signs and symptoms of which the woman has complained and for which she has been treated, the record is vulnerable to an ongoing reconstruction as part of a narrative designed to sway or convince a jury. In a courtroom, in front of a jury, all of the woman's medical history becomes relevant, dating to her infancy and childhood. The record is combed for information that will buttress either the plaintiff's claim that she was healthy until she got implants, after which her health declined, or the defense's claim that she was, instead, always unhealthy and her current maladies were simply a continuation of an ongoing series of illnesses. The record is searched for clues that relate to her particular current problems, as well as items that might speak to her moral character, such as abortions, miscarriages, smoking, drinking, or violence.

The record in this case does not serve as a factual outline of the woman's medical history, but as a weapon in the legal battle being waged. The power of this weapon derives in large part from the fact that it can be interpreted and reconstructed. Berger and Luckmann (1967) describe the reconstruction of biography, a process in which we all engage, allowing us to bring the events of the past into conformity with the present. He suggests that whether we are college professors or prostitutes, we selectively comb our past, targeting events and experiences that help us make sense of the present, which account for our path from then to now. In a similar fashion, the plaintiff or victim in court is reconstructed through the use of formal or official information as well as through other associations. In court, women with implants discover that their entire history, gathered incrementally and haphazardly, is placed into patterns of meaning by the attorneys on both sides of a case.

No direct relationship exists between the medical record that is developed in the doctor's office and relied on heavily in court by both plaintiff and defendant as legal evidence and the reality presented by the women themselves. At best, the record can only approximate the symptoms reported, and at worst, it is diced into bits and pieces whose meaning is reconstructed in court, apart from the framework of meaning in which it was established. The interaction that is recorded is viscous, palpable, and organic, but the record is inert, accepted in its rigidified form as fact. The facts are constructed during presentation to the jury as a narrative to tell either the defense's or the plaintiff's story. In this process, there may be only a vague similarity between the meaning that entered the production of the record and the meaning that is reconstructed for presentation.

An excerpt from one trial transcript illustrates not only the process of construction of the record, but also the redoubled effort to reconstruct it during examination of the plaintiff. The defense attorney questions the doctor regarding complications experienced by a woman with implants:

Q: Who told the patient to stop playing golf?

A: [She] did. [She decided to quit.]

Q: Because of her dizziness?

A: Well, I don't know if it was because of her dizziness. I think she was complaining more of the fatigue, if I remember correctly.

Q: Take a look at your report.

A: It may be—I mean, I may have said it, but I think the main reason she stopped playing golf is because of the fatigue. Maybe the reason she stopped skiing was because of the dizziness and fear of falling.

Q: Have you reviewed her medical or other records to indicate whether the dizziness, in fact, began at that time period?

A: Well, there's some question. I think she told one of the other examiners that her dizziness started five years ago. When I looked through her records looking for dizziness occurrences or complaints of tilt or unsteadiness, I did not see any consistent pattern, so I really couldn't draw any conclusions. . . . The problem with relying on a spatial disorientation history is typically the physicians ignore the complaints or don't put them down and don't explore them. (*Jennings v. Baxter*, 1995)

This example illustrates the efforts of one party to rely on a record as a statement of fact, and the other, the doctor being cross-examined, to demonstrate that it may actually not reflect fact, while still trying to preserve his status as a competent professional.

The attorneys fully acknowledge the medical record as a social construction through the way they use it. They piece together different parts of the record, imbuing them with meaning that would not be possible if the record simply reflected some objective reality, a preexisting truth. The manner in which medical records are used in the courtroom indicates a recognition of the problematic assumption of objectivity of medical records, while at the same time, insisting on their value precisely because of their purported factual status. Both sides, while developing a meaningful narrative based on the medical records to present to a jury, present this narrative as fact rather than as a result of a reconstruction of what was even at its inception a negotiated construction.

In a 1995 case in federal court, 3M, while admitting that the plaintiff was very sick and dying, insisted that the medical records revealed a person who was a liar, a person who should not be believed, because she had told even her own doctors different things at different times. For example, she had denied having a baby at one point, when in fact she had a child she had given up. In addition, she did not tell the truth about how much she smoked and for how long. The defense asserted that her physical problems were a result of smoking. The record was used for several purposes. First, to build a definition of the plaintiff as sick, but sick as a result of something other than silicone poisoning or autoimmune disease. Second, the record was used to establish her character or, in this case, to tarnish it by finding discrepancies between what she says, what her deposition reports, and what is contained in her medical records. Furthermore, through selective presentation of her record, she can be constructed as a malingerer or a hypochondriac rather than a legitimate patient.

The record in Charlotte Mahlum's case illustrates the defense using the medical records to characterize her as biologically deviant: having poor vision, starting her period at an exceptionally young age, developing precociously. This, they claimed, made her susceptible to auto-immune problems later on. Furthermore, when the plaintiff "opened the door" on posttraumatic stress syndrome, the defense relied on her records to introduce the fact that she had been battered by her husband. In addition, the defense tried to portray her as a hypochondriac, demonstrating with diagrams that she had been to the doctor over thirty times during the last ten years. Indeed, the plaintiff then turned this tactic back on itself, establishing that she had gone on the average three times a year, and this was inclusive of the periods of surgery and recovery. In fact, then, she was a very infrequent and sometimes reluctant patient.

This creative process is fascinating to watch in court, and its consequences are potentially devastating or redeeming to the client. Much depends on the artfulness of the argument attorneys can present, as well as the jury's ability to assess the different presentations of reality.

Charlotte Mahlum's examination by the plaintiff attorney, Ernest Hornsby, and the cross-examination by the attorney for Dow Chemical Company, Don Nomura, illustrate the process through which records are used to construct contradictory realities. For the plaintiff:

Hornsby: You sat in here the last two and a half, three weeks and you've heard the doctors talk about your health?

Mahlum: Yes, I have.

Hornsby: Just like we all have. And I want to ask you a couple of questions about prior to 1985. I want to get to that in a minute. You got your breast implants in 1985?

Mahlum: Yes.

Hornsby: But prior to that time, going back to your medical records, you had gallbladder surgery, I believe in 1974?

Mahlum: Yes, I did.

Hornsby: At the same time they took your gallbladder out in 1974 they also removed your appendix?

Mahlum: Yes.

Hornsby: And there was a tubal done; is that right?

Mahlum: Yes.

Hornsby: Were you having some gallbladder problems and some symptoms prior to 1974 that led up to a diagnosis of having your gallbladder removed?

Mahlum: Yes, I was. I was having pains in like my arms and in my stomach area.

Hornsby: And did the doctors diagnose gallbladder as the cause of your problems?

Mahlum: Yes, they did.

Hornsby: They removed your gallbladder?

Mahlum: Yes.

Hornsby: Did the problems return?

Mahlum: No, they went away after I healed up from the surgeries.

Hornsby: In 1983 I believe you had a hiatal hernia diagnosed?

Mahlum: Yes, I did. I had gone to one doctor and he had suggested that I have an EKG, which I did. He figured I was having a heart attack because of the pains in my chest and arms. I had doctors tell me I had ulcers. They were prescribing ulcer medication, which didn't do nothing. And, I went to Dr. Giltner in Minot, and I told him my problems. He said I'll bet you've got a hiatal hernia. We did surgery. He repaired it for me, and that took care of the problems.

Hornsby: The hiatal hernia problems that you had you said was burning in your chest?

Mahlum: Yes, it was, it was right up here underneath my breast bone. And he told me I would not know the difference between a heart attack or the hiatal hernia, it was the same symptoms.

Hornsby: So, now in '74 you had the gallbladder out. And in '83, I take it for some time prior to that you were having these heart attack symptoms of a hiatal hernia; is that right?

Mahlum: Yes, I was.

Hornsby: And one doctor misdiagnosed it?

Mahlum: Yes.

Hornsby: He told you you were having a heart attack?

Mahlum: Yes.

Hornsby: Then Dr. Giltner figured out what the problem was, right?

Mahlum: Yes.

Hornsby: And repaired the hiatal hernia?

Mahlum: Yes.

Hornsby: Were you having any more problems from those symptoms you were having before that?

Mahlum: No, I didn't.

Then followed a discussion about the fact that Charlotte Mahlum had suffered frostbite while living in North Dakota. Continuing:

Hornsby: And the two childbirths you had were all normal; is that right?

Mahlum: Yes, they were.

Hornsby: We've heard testimony from the doctors who have testified here who have both examined you and looked at your records. They've also looked through your medical records to determine if there was anything there that they could spot that seemed to be some type of a start of a disease process or whatever. And their testimony, of course, was that they had not seen anything. But I want to ask you, do you recall in your health, prior to 1985 when you got your implants, that you had anything, any disease or any condition other than what we've just talked about here?

Mahlum: I would have your typical cold, flu, like everyone else. But just as soon as they would give me some antibiotic to clear it up, I would be fine again.

Hornsby: Now, in 1984, you had a rather frightening occurrence happen; isn't that right? You found a lump in your breast. (*Mahlum v. Dow Chemical*, 1995:127–131)

The questioning then moved into the area of her decision to have a mastectomy after the doctor found precancerous cells, and the subsequent surgeries. I present this rather lengthy interaction to demonstrate the construction of a biography of a healthy, normal woman. Now, to contrast this with the interaction between Charlotte Mahlum and the attorney for Dow Chemical, Mr. Nomura, who relies on the medical record to paint a picture of an abnormally developed female:

Nomura: Now, I notice that you're wearing glasses today. How long or what age were you when you first started wearing glasses?

Mahlum: I was three.

Nomura: At age three?

Mahlum: Yes.

Nomura: And you've been, I guess, wearing them since that early age in life?

Mahlum: Yes, I have.

Nomura: And, you're nearsighted? Farsighted?

Mahlum: Nearsighted.

Nomura: Are they corrected to 20–20?

Mahlum: Yes—well, if I remember right on my prescription I think they're only corrected to like 20–40.

Nomura: When was the last time that you saw your optometrist for your lens corrections, I guess?

Mahlum: I think it was '93.

Nomura: But you haven't been back to the optometrist since then for any type of lens adjustment then?

Mahlum: I went to the eye doctor, Dr. Miller, down there at U. C. Davis.

Nomura: I recall 1993.

Mahlum: And he told me that my glasses were fine.

Nomura: Since that time you haven't sought additional optometry care for your glasses?

Mahlum: I went to a eye doctor here in town, but he did not do a checkup.

Nomura: Did other people in your family have eyeglasses as early as age three that they needed it, your brothers, sisters, that type of thing?

Mahlum: No.

Nomura: Did they need glasses at all or is that something that came up later in life for them?

Mahlum: Most of them were later years.

Nomura: Another thing, and again I apologize for being somewhat personal, but there's a lot of things that have been asked of you and a lot of things I suppose that need to be asked of you. But do you recall when you would have had your first period, when menses first occurred for you?

Mahlum: Yes, I think it was when I was nine.

Nomura: Nine years old?

Mahlum: Yes.

Nomura: And you have a sister, do you not?

Mahlum: Yes.

Nomura: More than just one or just one?

Mahlum: I have three.

Nomura: And did your sisters have menses or their period at such an early age, nine years of age?

Mahlum: No, they did not.

Nomura: Did they have it more like 13, 14?

Mahlum: Two of them did and one had her's start at about 16, if I remember right.

Nomura: So at least in a couple of areas, then, the glasses and the menses, your medical history was a little different than your siblings, then, back when you were children, at least in those couple of areas?

Mahlum: I don't know if you would call that different. Some people wear glasses early in life.

Nomura: I don't mean different from the population at large. It was just different from what your sisters and brothers, their particular situation?

Mahlum: Yes.

Here followed a discussion of her household situation. The next questioning related to records continued:

Nomura: Now, in the time period before August of 1985, in July of 1985 when the implant, the mastectomy occurred and the implant occurred, you lived predominantly for the preceding ten years in the Dakotas?

Mahlum: Yes, we did.

Nomura: In the Kenmare area?

Mahlum: Yes.

Nomura: And in the Kenmare area, again this is probably 1974, 1975 through 1985, you had occasion to see doctors as needed, to go to the emergency room or go to see a physician if you needed any particular medical care, did you not?

Mahlum: Yes.

Nomura: And looking at your records, independent of the birth of your two children, which required medical care, there were, I counted it up, to be roughly somewhere in the neighborhood of 35 to 40 visits to the Kenmare Clinic or to the ER room or to a physician in that ten-year period between 1974 and 1985. Does that generally comport with your memory or recall?

Mahlum: No, I would never think there was that many. Because I am not one to go to the doctor unless I feel that there's a very big necessity.

Nomura: Let me ask it in this fashion then, ma'am. Did you go to the doctor in 1974 through August of 1985, and again I'm sorry, July, July and August of 1985. I'm talking about the time period, just so we can have a segmented area for you and for the jury, that between 1974 and when you found out that you had fibrocystic disease and found out that doctors recommended that you have both breasts removed, that's the time period that I'm referring to now?

Mahlum: I would remember that I went like for colds, that they would give me antibiotics, or like flu type, but nothing serious.

Nomura: That's what I'm referring to. In that time period, between 1974 and when you had this problem with the fibrocystic disease and the need for the mastectomy, did you go to the doctor for things like coughs and colds?

Mahlum: Occasionally.

Nomura: So that you could get some treatment for maladies or illnesses that were relatively minor?

Mahlum: Yes. (*Mahlum v. Dow Chemical*, 1995:179–195)

Mr. Nomura continues for the next nine pages of the transcript with questions designed to show the jury that Charlotte Mahlum was not reluctant to seek medical care when she had minor ailments, such as bone spurs or a sprained ankle. He also tries to demonstrate that she had experienced urinary incontinence and swollen joints prior to having implants in 1985. Building on this background, he then questions her in a manner designed to convince the jury that if she had been experiencing fatigue and pain after having her implants, as she has said she did, she would have sought medical attention; yet, she did not. A sequence of Mr. Nomura's questions is presented to illustrate this point:

In 1987, when you went in for bone spurs, did you discuss with your physicians at that time this generalized weakness, this strength that had left your body?

In 1991, you went to the doctor four or five times for the sprained ankle. . . . did you discuss with him any of the symptoms that you described as having arisen in 1990 and 1991?

Did you see doctors in 1990 for these symptoms you've described in court?

Did you see doctors in 1988 or '89 or '86 or '87 for this strength or weakness whatsoever you described?

And in 1992 did you see any doctors for these symptoms that had begun as early as 1985, some in 1990 and some in 1991, that persisted?

So the couple doctors you did see in this eight-year period, you did not mention these symptoms to, correct? (*Mahlum v. Dow Chemical*, 1995)

This line of questioning continues, building the case that Mrs. Mahlum must not have been suffering the symptoms she discussed in court if she didn't mention them to doctors in these several instances.

The record, while important, and in fact while determining for some juries, is open not just to interpretation, but to manipulation and re-creation. As important as it is, however, it is the record of only one woman and her medical experience. To make the case not just that the woman is sick, but that she is sick because of silicone leakage in her system, requires that the plaintiff first show through evidence acceptable to the judge that silicone can cause autoimmune disease. This very important issue is at the heart of the debate about "junk science" and real science. In the following chapter, we turn to these concerns and to the significant debates about science, and the relationship between science and evidence.

9

The Medical-Legal Controversy and Its Impact on Litigation

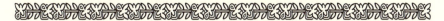

> As the primary custodians of individual rights, courts [are] sensitized to threats posed by science and technology to individual safety and autonomy.
> —Sheila Jasanoff quoted in *Blum v. Merrell Dow*, 1996

In breast implant litigation, the fight for admissibility of evidence is one of the most important and most hotly contested battles attorneys wage. The jury, as the decider of fact, can only decide on the "facts" if they are introduced and admitted into evidence. These facts are not introduced directly by attorneys but instead through witnesses, often expert witnesses. Witnesses called by either side can testify about any number of items related to breast implant cases, such as the estimated long-term cost of unemployment or disability, the medical, mental, and social history of the plaintiff, the amount and type of knowledge held or disclaimed by the defendant, as well as scientific findings about implants and their relationship to disease. In certain cases, scientific evidence must be approved in advance by the judge, whose gatekeeping role is of major significance in cases built around scientific research.

In breast implant litigation, in some jurisdictions, and always in federal court, the judge's assessment of the validity of scientific methodologies and their decisions regarding admissibility of scientific evidence can establish the battle plan for plaintiff and defendant. Before the case goes to trial, many of the important decisions about evidence and experts have already been made. What the jury then gets to evaluate is often severely curtailed by these pre-trial decisions. There has been lively discussion about the trial judge's gatekeeping function, with many scholars seeing it as subject to abuse and as an unfair usurpation of the jury's right to decide the facts. Others, primarily from the defense side, sound alarms about the jury's inability to distinguish science from hoopla.

The troublesome relationship between science and the introduction of scientific evidence in the courtroom needs to be clarified. The discrepancy between the purpose and method of science and the purpose and method of litigation is illustrated in the courtroom when experts and attorneys rely on the interpretation of scientific findings, but do so with very different assumptions and understandings. As a result, the expert's opinion and testimony often has a different meaning for the expert than it does for the attorney and the jury. Discussions of such basic methodological terms as sampling, means, averages and medians, confidence levels, and normal curves are likely to be interpreted differently by experts and others in court. The unavoidable difference between the way scientists understand science and the way judges and jurors understand science, as well as the problems this presents when judges and jurors are asked to make decisions about difficult scientific debates, shapes the important decision-making processes that take place in the courtroom.

Perhaps the clearest example of the different meanings of the same question is in the very basic query: does A (silicone) cause B (diseases) in some women? In a court of law, the burden of proof is on the plaintiff breast implant victim to show that it is *more likely than not* that silicone was a substantial factor in causing the woman's disease. For example, even if the jury finds it only 51 percent likely that silicone caused the disease and 49 percent likely that it did not, the woman wins her case because it is *probable* that silicone caused the harm, even if it is possible that it did not. The reason for this is simple: if plaintiffs, to prove their case, had to wait until science and medicine reached a 95 percent certainty that silicone caused the disease, that could be waiting decades. This is, by the way, the suggestion of Marcia Angell in her book, *Science on Trial* (1996). However, since "justice delayed is justice denied," civil courts allow the jury to make common-sense determinations based on the weight of the *presently available evidence*, if that evidence points to probable causation.

In the studies that the manufacturers rely on to show no "causation," the authors of the studies require proof to a 95 percent certainty before they will conclude that a cause and effect relationship exists between silicone and disease. When science is used in the courtroom, judges and juries must understand the difference between causation as acceptable among researchers and causation as acceptable within the courtroom. The necessity for judges to make decisions about admissibility of scientific evidence must allow for an acknowledgment of the severe restrictions applied to the finding of "cause" in scientific research.

The debate about the facts of silicone breast implants and their relationship to connective tissue disease and other diseases, as well as the debate about the interpretations of the scientific studies that address this relationship, is loud and strong. This debate is at the center of women's efforts to be compensated by manufacturers for the pain and suffering they experience from implants. Although we have addressed the studies related to such problems as gel bleed, rupture, inertness of silicone, silicone migration, and the effects of silicone on the human body elsewhere, here let us briefly summarize the main problems related to implants.

Capsular contracture, the building of a fibrous scar tissue in response to an inflammation provoked by the introduction of a foreign substance into the body, is a frequent and anticipated problem, occurring in about half of all implant cases (Angell, 1996). The closed capsulotomy used to break the scar tissue apart may well rupture the implant, spilling the silicone into the body and carrying it through the bloodstream and lymph channels to other parts of the body.

Another problem clearly associated with implants is silicone leakage or "bleed," or "sweat," in which silicone escapes from the pores of the gel-filled implant and migrates across the tissue planes and through the bloodstream to other organs. If silicone were inert, this would be a much different situation than if it affects the organs and tissues to which it migrates. Because all implants bleed, the impact of silicone gel on the tissues and organs is of great significance.

Local reactions indicate that silicone gel is not as "biocompatible" as some physicians have thought. Rather, the body considers the gel as harmful and offensive. It mobilizes giant macrophages, a type of white blood cell that forms in reaction to foreign bodies such as implants, and tries to "eat" the silicone implant, causing inflammation (Vasey and Feldstein, 1993). However, the macrophages cannot "digest" the silicone particles like they can other foreign invaders. Thus, they continue to attack the silicone without success, and the body's immune system remains constantly alert, trying to dispose of something that it cannot. This process is called autoimmune disease or immune system dysfunction.

The fact that implants could rupture has long been widely accepted by manufacturers and researchers, just as they have been aware of other significant problems. The rate of rupture estimates vary widely, with manufacturers significantly under-representing both the rate of ruptures and their knowledge of problems (U.S. Congress, 1993). Robinson et al. (1995) concludes that roughly 63.5% of the breast implants that have been in place between one and twenty-five years rupture or leak. Vasey and

Feldstein point out that whether they rupture within a year or after twenty years, almost all implants will eventually rupture. D. L. de Camara shows a "positive correlation between the number of leaking and ruptured silicone gel implants and the duration of implantation time." In her study of fifty-one silicone gel implants, all implants older than 10 years were ruptured or leaking silicone gel (1993).

The newer, thinner implants rupture more easily than the older, thicker ones, and most have no obvious rupture cause. The rates of implant disruption (overt rupture or bleed severe enough to string out over 12 inches) were similar with and without symptoms (72% and 71%, respectively), a finding which led Robinson and his colleagues to advocate prophylactic removal of breast implants within 8 years of implantation (Brown et al., 1997).

Yet another problem is the difficulties presented to mammography by implants. The implant often obstructs the passage of X rays through the tissue, resulting in the possibility of a delayed detection of cancer (Handel et al., 1993). Thus, women with breast implants may be less likely to be diagnosed with breast cancer at an early and treatable stage, although digital mammography may be superior to conventional mammography for cancer assessment (Brown et al., 1997). Other concerns are the possible rupture of the implant during mammography, and the failure of mammography to detect a rupture in the implant. Even ultrasonagraphy is likely to not detect a significant number of ruptured implants (Brown, et al., 1997).

One question presented to jurors in their decision making is whether the woman was aware of these potential problems. Did she make an informed choice after being told of all the major potential and actual risks and consequences? We have noted that, especially in cases of implants for augmentation, jurors can be unduly harsh with a woman who was willing to take a chance with her body. Although the immunology community was aware of significant problems, twenty or twenty-five years ago no lay woman, to her great misfortune, had heard of any dangers associated with implants, either from her doctor or from the media (Stewart and Ross, 1996). In very few cases were women told anything of possible negative consequences. Most physicians, passing on the weak warnings of manufacturers in the package inserts, even failed to warn of predictable local complications.

Informed consent is one thing, but uninformed consent is quite another. Yet, even if the woman had consented to a potentially dangerous surgery for a condition that was not life threatening, would she have known the true impact silicone might have on her body? The most likely answer is "no." She would have had no reports from manufacturers that there were any problems, her doctor would not have warned her, and she would have confidently sought the surgery, with no expectation of problems. Although there were several hundred articles on breast implants, especially on their medical and biological properties, women had no reason to go to their medical school library and peruse the scientific and medical literature. Unfortunately, plastic surgeons weren't interested either. Women responded in the same way most of us do when seeking medical care: they asked their doctors and trusted the response.

Plastic surgeons and manufacturers successfully fought the FDA's efforts to require that all implant patients receive a brochure on the safety of implants. More recently, they successfully altered the FDA's initial statements of risk which were included on the informed consent form available to women who were permitted implants, those in the "urgent need" category or "open availability" protocol (those with mastectomies or serious deformities). Manufacturers were aware of significant potential problems with implants and implant gel, and suspected a relationship between the many symptoms of nonclassical connective tissue disease and silicone gel implants. Yet, trying to maintain their market as well as protect themselves against liability, they argued against their own suspicions and knowledge, insisting that breast implants were not associated with connective tissue disease. They further argued that if indeed there was an association, they, the manufacturers, should not be held responsible because they had informed the doctors of potential problems. Even those feeble warnings offered by manufacturers in their package inserts were watered down by the salespeople in the field. Dow Corning, while acknowledging in its package inserts that there were "reports of suspected immunological responses to silicone mammary implants," also asserted that a "review of the published experimental findings and clinical experience shows that convincing evidence does not exist to support a causal relationship between exposure to silicone materials and the acquisition of or exacerbation of a variety of rheumatic and connective tissue disorders" (Angell, 1996:57). Yet, Hennekens et al. (1996) shows a 30 percent increase of autoimmune problems among women with implants.

Dow Corning and the other manufacturers were sidestepping the question, "Were breast implants safe?" Quite simply, despite the fact that hundreds of thousands of these devices had been placed in women's bodies, the question of safety had not been addressed. Plastic surgeons were *assuming* safety, and manufacturers weren't revealing what they suspected. FDA Commissioner Kessler, as late as 1991, twenty-five years after these devices were implanted in women by the thousands, called the lack of data produced by manufacturers on the safety of implants "appalling" (Angell, 1996:55). He concluded that the manufacturers had failed to produce reasonable assurances of the safety and effectiveness of silicone gel breast implants.

Plaintiffs' lawyers were able in a number of jury cases to point out that manufacturers had inadequate safety information about the products they were selling. More than that, they also had reason to suspect problems which they ignored and had hard evidence of problems which they hid. In court, this sort of evidence was coupled with evidence that a woman was severely ill and with testimony from toxicologists and rheumatologists that there were autoimmune responses to silicone and that silicone traveled throughout the body. This convinced some juries that the manufacturer had responsibility for the woman's illness, and further that the manufacturer should pay punitive damages for its conscious disregard of human safety.

The two major aspects of a successful lawsuit are liability and causation. Juries routinely find liability on the part of the corporations based on their corporate conduct. But that is not enough. The jury must also find that the manufacturers' bad conduct *caused* harm to the woman. Naturally, the corporations and the injured women disagree about causation, specifically about the impact of silicone gel on the body, both directly through local reactions and through systemic autoimmune responses.

Questions of causation are central to the case. The jury, as the decider of fact, is placed in the position of assessing all of the relevant research and clinical experience that is admitted and determining whether there is a 51 percent probability that the product, in this case breast implants, caused the illness or harm. There is enormous controversy in this area, and it is here that the methodologies that are used in conducting research become significant to the admissibility of evidence to the jury. The defense's position is that proof of a causal relationship between silicone breast implants and autoimmune diseases has not been established; hence, these cases should not even go to a jury. The plaintiff's position is that there is a strong probability, given all of the evidence available, that a causal connection exists between silicone breast implants and autoimmune disease, and a jury should be allowed to hear all the evidence, weigh it, and make a decision.

THE *DAUBERT* DECISION

The question about what evidence is admissible in court is enormously important. Most jurors remain unaware of the extensive decision making that goes on outside their presence regarding admissibility. The weekend, the evening, and the early morning conferences, crucial for the proceedings of the day (as well as for building a record in the event of an appeal), determine much of what the jurors will hear and see. The published rules of evidence and the judge's interpretation of these rules, as well as the rulings made by that judge, provide the framework for the case, thereby making issues of admissibility the skeleton on which the arguments are built.

The relatively new, and on its face more liberal, standard resulting from *Daubert v. Merrell Dow Pharmaceuticals* (1993) has replaced *Frye*, which became the standard for admissibility of evidence in federal cases in 1923. The *Frye* standard allowed only that evidence meet the criterion of "general acceptability in the field," thereby minimizing the admissibility of "junk science" by requiring that scientific evidence be based on "principles and methods generally accepted in the scientific community." Its opponents claimed that it would limit novel ideas and findings. For example, Galileo's testimony that the earth revolved around the sun or Columbus' assertion that the earth was round, flying in the face of generally accepted knowledge, would have been inadmissible. *Frye* also severely constrained the jury's role in deciding the facts. The *Frye* standard, however, was not used in all courts, nor was it universally accepted. In fact, during the seventy years after *Frye* was decided, the Supreme Court did not once cite *Frye* in a majority decision until the *Daubert* decision. Furthermore, the Supreme Court has studiously avoided making a major statement about the role of science in the law (Walker and Monahan, 1996).

In 1975, President Gerald Ford signed into law new Rules of Evidence establishing criteria for the admissibility of expert testimony, which included Federal Rule 702, requiring scientific validity, thus the evidentiary *relevance* and *reliability* of the proposed submission. This rule omitted the requirement for "general acceptance in the scientific community"; instead, it made "evidentiary reliability . . . based on scientific validity" the standard in cases involving scientific evidence (Walker and Monahan, 1996:844). Federal courts interpreted the new Rules differently, with some courts using one standard and some the other. The result was a somewhat inconsistent response to a rapidly changing scientific world. In 1993, the U.S. Supreme Court, in reversing the Ninth Circuit, tackled the question of what constituted expert testimony, finally addressing the question of the criteria that constitute science which can be admitted, and held that the Federal Rules supersede Frye. This, however, did not allow for the admissibility of all expert testimony. Rather, where a genuine dispute occurs, federal judges are now given the power to conduct a preliminary *Daubert* hearing in which they assess the reasoning and methodology underlying the testimony to determine its validity, relevance, and admissibility. Walker and Monahan (1996) suggest that *Daubert* "heralds a new receptivity to science in law ... a new openness to the fruits of the scientific method" (838–839).

The *Daubert* standard, reflecting Federal Rule 702, allows much greater latitude than was allowed by *Frye* in the introduction of expert testimony. It is still designed to keep away from the jury totally unfounded or ludicrous points of view. Because it acknowledges that, for a variety of reasons, conclusions not shared by the majority of the medical or scientific community are not necessarily wrong, the judge is sometimes placed in the position of being the "gatekeeper." Rather than focus on findings and outcomes, the *Daubert* decision requires that the methodology of the study be scientifically reliable before it is admitted. Thus, two studies and two expert opinions reaching opposite conclusions would both be admissible under *Daubert* as long as the methodology used to arrive at these conclusions was valid. If the research or the expert opinion is methodologically sound, then it should be allowed even if the conclusions are so novel or so unexpected that they fly in the face of generally accepted medical knowledge. In *Daubert*, the defense, on appeal, convinced the Supreme Court that novel medical information and findings can be valid and reliable. They did this through the introduction of epidemiological studies which supported their position that there was no connection between Bendectin and birth defects. Interestingly, while this case used epidemiological studies to support novel findings, epidemiology is used in the research on breast implants to convince judges that only the most conservative interpretations of science are acceptable.

As a result of the *Daubert* decision, judges were asked to evaluate the validity and reliability of the methodology through which scientific or medical evidence is generated before that evidence could be introduced to the jurors through expert testimony. Judges, often with no more scientific expertise than laypeople, were suddenly thrust into the position of being asked to evaluate very sophisticated methodological questions, and at least indirectly, to evaluate the legitimacy and validity of research findings on which the case made by plaintiffs and defendants rested. Judges were now, more than ever, placed in the position of being criticized for their decisions about admissibility. Clearly, the parties in these cases shortly after *Daubert*, judges as well as attorneys, recognized that they were feeling their way through new and untested legal waters. One of the reasons Judge Jones's decision in *Hall v. Baxter*, has been so closely watched by the legal community is because he relied on a panel of experts to assess the *Daubert* testimony.

In evaluating the methodology of the research on which the expert was to testify, the judge is expected to evaluate a process about which scientists themselves may disagree. When trial court judges have gone too far, in keeping scientific evidence they disagreed with away from the jury (as is probably the case in the December 18, 1996 case heard by Judge Robert Jones in Oregon), these decisions have often been over-turned by appellate courts and criticized in legal journals. Judges have also been condemned for purportedly allowing "junk science" into their courtroom in more than one case. In the *Mahlum* case, for example, Judge Connie Steinheimer was subjected to a manufacturer-orchestrated trashing by the *Wall Street Journal*, the *New York Times*, and numerous other papers for allegedly allowing "junk science" into the courtroom, thereby permitting the plaintiffs to convince a "naive jury" that implants were dangerous. An editorial in the *Wall Street Journal* on November 8, 1995 accused: "What happened in this case is what's happened in other breast implant cases: The judge refused to act as a gatekeeper against pseudo-scientific testimony—a role spelled out by most state supreme courts and the U.S. Supreme Court's 1993 *Daubert v. Merrell Dow* decision." The editorial continues, suggesting that the plaintiff's bar has bought off the judges: "The judge's reluctance to police the plaintiff's bar should hardly be surprising. A study by the American Tort Reform Association found that in three of the most plaintiff-friendly states—Alabama, California, and Texas—the trial lawyers contributed $17.3 million to political candidates, including many judges, between 1990 and 1994" (*Wall Street Journal*, November 8, 1995:A18).

Such editorializing is a muddled jumble of misinterpretation and misinformation, condemnations that read like press releases from the corporations, and that are accepted and printed without question by very influential newspapers. Perhaps the corporate status of both the manufacturers and the newspapers leads to such unquestioning acceptance by the press. The press has been vulnerable to severe criticisms in the breast implant litigation for allowing itself to be "spoon-fed" false and misleading information by the manufacturers and printing it without scrutiny as if it were fact (F.A.I.R., January–February 1996).

Following the Mahlum trial, a letter to the editor asserted that the judge's decision to allow plaintiffs to introduce the scientific evidence they did would "put these political, obviously biased individuals out of work at the next election" (Skogerson, 1995). While Judge Steinheimer handily won reelection in the post-Mahlum elections, vituperative attacks such as these surely did not go unnoticed by other judges in Nevada and elsewhere, not only in states where judges are elected, but also in federal courts.

Since 1993, a number of breast implant cases have been shaped by the

Daubert rules, for example: *Hopkins v. Dow Corning, Vasallo v. Baxter, Merlin v. 3M, Hall v. Baxter.* Under *Daubert,* various misunderstandings present themselves when we look at the role of scientific testimony in the courtroom. From transcripts of *Daubert* hearings as well as from personal observations of two hearings on admissibility, the following emerge as potential problems: (1) science is often perceived as a finished product, not a process; (2) few persons, except the expert witnesses, understand, or can be expected to understand, the subtleties of scientific methodology; (3) the terminology used by experts is misunderstood; (4) the whole manner in which scientific studies are conducted and the expectations we can reasonably have about these studies and their findings is deeply misunderstood by the judges and attorneys; (5) the subtleties and complexities of methodology as well as the relationship between theory, hypothesis, and research are misunderstood; (6) the relationship between the norm or average or curves and the individual case being considered is misunderstood; (7) the underlying purpose of research is often misunderstood; (8) the ability of any study to prove cause and effect is misunderstood, as is the relationship between cause and correlation; (9) judges and attorneys often assume science is a static set of agreed upon procedures rather than the dynamic and conflicted area of methodological and theoretical disagreements it is; (10) judges and attorneys may assume that there is *a* scientific method, when in fact there are many and there are many debates about the appropriateness of each in particular circumstances as well as the correctness of application of the methodology; and (11) much of the enterprise of science is the criticism of others' work—science is not only the pursuit of knowledge, but also the pursuit of power and status. Those engaged in this competitive activity have a great personal as well as professional stake in the ascendancy of their method.

One would not expect a nonscientist jury or judge to fully understand or appreciate the vagaries of different scientific methodologies or the limits or biases inherent in the methodology itself. But if scientific methodologies and data developed from scientific research are so crucial in the courtroom, then those persons who are relying on it or criticizing it should have at least some rudimentary knowledge of the scientific undertaking. Yet, as the following cases reveal, the parties, through no fault of their own, are often confused, and sometimes simply wrong in their interpretations. If *Daubert* is going to be allowed to take on such importance in our justice system, it seems only reasonable that those persons making the crucial decisions about admissibility should have some understanding of science, research, and methodology. To expect judges to make decisions deeply embedded in an understanding of science and methodology, deciding issues that belong to a jury is absurd. To do so confuses the purposes and rules of science with the purposes and rules of the courtroom. In addition, and perhaps more importantly, in our system of justice, the jury is the finder of fact. We must remember that. The jury sifts through the arguments and evidence and cross-examinations and summary comments of the attorneys under the watchful eye of the judge. The jury deliberates and decides. The black robes belong on the bench, not in the jury box.

A look at one breast implant trial in federal court in which the judge necessarily relied on the *Daubert* decision in establishing admissibility of scientific evidence reveals the extreme difficulties which the gatekeeping function presents not just to the judge but to the justice system. In the pre-trial "*Daubert* hearing" in the *Merlin v. 3M/McGhan* case, the focus was not on whether implants burst or became hard or lumpy or disfigured the breast, or caused maiming when removed. These problems were easy to establish without the necessity of a complex *Daubert* hearing. And although the *Daubert* hearing is supposed to be about methodology, arguing causation seems commonplace. The questions to be decided in the pre-trial hearing were both jury questions. First, can silicone gel-filled implants cause a particular constellation of symptoms and signs? Many of those symptoms are almost identical to classic diseases, but are found in a new configuration, which can comprise a new disease. Second, if so, did these implants cause these symptoms and diseases in the plaintiff? While the plaintiff contended that there was a new disease, caused by leaking silicone causing an autoimmune reaction, plaintiff also acknowledged that the science in this area was still emerging. The plaintiff maintained that there were many questions regarding the biological and toxicological interactions which cause the signs and symptoms they claimed were tied to silicone gel leakage.

It is crucial to the plaintiff that the jury find "causation," in addition to the liability (fault) claims against the manufacturer, such as fraud or misrepresentation. These two areas are often interrelated, so that the evidence that would show causation is often contained in the same research that has been fraudulently concealed from the public or the FDA. However, without the judge's decision to admit plaintiff's studies supporting a relationship between silicone gel and these signs and symptoms, based on the acceptability of their methodology, the case is over no matter how outrageous the liability is.

In *Merlin*, the defense contended that while the plaintiff was indeed ill, even dying, she was not sick as a result of implants. The defense claimed that there were no valid, reliable studies based on sound methodology which proved that implants cause illness. The defendants relied heavily on epidemiological studies, which concluded that there was no observed relationship between silicone gel and classic connective tissue disease to buttress their claim that they were not responsible for Mildred Merlin's illness, even if they knew of studies that indicated the dangers of silicone, its ability to migrate, and its lack of inertness. They based their defense on a couple of studies, which looked good with a cursory glance and which sounded convincing.

The interactions in court were negotiations in the construction of reality, as they always are. Both sides worked under the new standard of methodological soundness, which replaced the standard of "general medical acceptability," and constructed their arguments to show either that the methodology was acceptable or it was not. Plaintiffs introduced experts who claimed that clinical experience and emerging data suggested a causal relationship between silicone and inflammation or autoimmune response, more generally illness. Defendants claimed instead that while clinical signs and symptoms and speculation and opinion may *suggest* such a relationship, there was no presently known entity that comprised a disease caused by silicone gel. This is a process of "claims making" as Spector and Kitsuse (1992) would point out, with agents on each side of an issue making a claim that a particular "truth" exists and engaging in a struggle of wills and resources for control over the definition of reality. Here the "trier of fact," the jury, will hear the presentation of facts as they are allowed before them. This is dependent on the judge's ability to determine whether a reasonable methodology was used in the studies being presented or cited by the expert witnesses.

An example of the lack of understanding of the use of statistics in scientific inquiry and interpretation was presented in the *Daubert* hearing for the *Merlin v. 3M/McGhan* case heard by Judge Howard McKibben in federal court in Nevada, on December 11, 1995. An expert for the plaintiff, Dr. Arthur Brawer, for illustrative purposes presented a graph of a curve representing the progress of the disease, which increases systematically during the first five years and then exponentially after that time. He discussed the curve as based on the average appearance of different disease symptoms at different times. Fatigue is one of the earliest signs for the average woman with breast implants, appearing at around two years, while cognitive dysfunction appears later, with approximately three-quarters of the women developing it after seven years, and with most affected women having a fully established disease after twelve years. Dr. Brawer pointed out that there is a good deal of variability in this disease, depending on such factors as the woman's health history, the length of time she had implants, what the fluid materials were, her susceptibility to silicone and disease, whether they burst or leaked, if so how long they had been ruptured, and other considerations. In court, the defense and the judge had a difficult time accepting the fact that Dr. Brawer could not place Mrs. Merlin exactly on the curve; that he could not simply list her symptoms, their date of appearance, and reflect the average of which the curve consisted. It seemed difficult to differentiate the normal from the average and to distinguish an individual case from a graph that reflected an averaging of hundreds of cases. Dr. Brawer was expected to demonstrate that Mildred Merlin's symptoms exactly mirrored the curve. The Judge wondered how a curve could be developed which reflected three hundred women, and Mrs. Merlin could not be placed accurately on it. Dr. Brawer's verbal skills were sorely challenged in his efforts to convince the judge that no one case would be expected to exactly mimic the average, and to assure him that did not mean Mrs. Merlin was therefore not suffering from silicone-related disease.

In *Jennings v. Baxter* (1995) in Oregon, Dr. Stuart Silverman for the plaintiffs had a similar problem communicating the difference between the norm and the individual case. He concluded: "we're dealing with people who have different genetics, who have different exposures and have different chemical exposures, one would expect a variety of responses." Part of the difficulty has to do with the similarity between many of the symptoms of silicone-related diseases and other classical connective tissue diseases, such as lupus, scleroderma, or chronic fatigue, and with the variability in the presentation of the symptoms that do form a pattern. About one-third appear early, one-third appear late, and one-third present themselves in a random fashion. Furthermore, since some researchers suggest that the silicone starts a reactive process that continues long after the implants are removed, it is possible that new symptoms appear in about 10 percent of the cases even after the removal of the implants (*Merlin v. 3M/McGhan*, 1996). Such a phenomenon disturbs the elegance of a straight-line cause and effect relationship.

The defense pushes for a definitive set of symptoms and signs that operate in a consistent manner across individuals, and that can be separated entirely from other similar or even related diseases and are unique to silicone breast-implanted women. Their goal in court and in evidentiary hearings is to convince the judge or jury that if the disease cannot be certainly established as a unique disease sharing no features with other similar diseases, it does not exist. In the *Mahlum* (1995) case, for example, the defense's first tactic was to try to convince the jury that silicone did not cause problems. Even if it did, the defense maintained that it had not caused Charlotte Mahlum's problems, which were instead problems of chronic fatigue or stress related to her relationships or childhood experiences. The plaintiff, on the other hand, recognizing that many symptoms are related to the autoimmune diseases caused by silicone gel breast implants which are similar to other ailments, had the task of convincing the jury that indeed this was a separate disease or illness that shares many characteristics of others. But because of the configuration, the number, or the relationship between symptoms, they constitute a separate disease caused by a foreign body reaction to silicone seepage into the tissues and bloodstream.

The plaintiffs' difficult task is made more difficult by the way in which the multidistrict litigation or "global settlement" disease grid was structured. For example, Dr. Brawer, was making the case that Mildred Merlin had an atypical autoimmune disease and that there was a constellation of different symptoms of which this new disease consisted. Dr. Brawer, however, had placed Mrs. Merlin in the category of scleroderma, leading Judge McKibben to query whether indeed this was a new disease then, or simply scleroderma. If it was new, then why had she been classified as having scleroderma? A close reading of the compensation category reveals that "The application of these diagnostic criteria is not intended to exclude from the compensation program individuals who present clinical symptoms or laboratory findings atypical of classical systemic sclerosis but who nonetheless have a systemic sclerosis-like (scleroderma-like) disease" (Breast Implant Litigation Settlement Agreement, March 29, 1994: 1). One disease category is for scleroderma, and when Dr. Brawer placed Mrs. Merlin on the grid, he included her in the category "Systemic Sclerosis/Scleroderma" (which is one of the compensation categories). The judge's question then was, if she had this new disease, why was she placed in the scleroderma category?

Dr. Brawer's response speaks to the intricate interface between science and law. To paraphrase: as a clinician who did not develop the grid, but was forced to work within its confines, he had to force his evaluations into categories that didn't fully reflect Mildred Merlin's symptoms. Brawer said that the grid was a testimony to the difficulty of getting women with a disease into categories that emerge from classic autoimmune diseases when they suffer atypical autoimmune diseases. The grid was developed by a committee of lawyers, with medical input, during a lengthy and complex settlement process, and not by doctors who actually see patients. Because the disease is legally defined, then the patients who are being assessed have to conform for settlement purposes to the legal definitions.

Judge McKibben, approaching the question somewhat differently, straightforwardly asked whether Mrs. Merlin had scleroderma or a new disease. If she didn't have scleroderma, why did Dr. Brawer identify her as having scleroderma on the settlement grid? Dr. Brawer responded from another direction, saying that identification of scleroderma is just a beginning point. Judge McKibben, understandably looking for certainty and predictability, asked whether the disease was so variable that we can't tell what it is. Defense followed with questions about why the American Society of Rheumatologists (ASR) had not distinguished criteria for this new disease. How, they asked, can there be 128 total symptoms that are tied to it? Defense demanded that Dr. Brawer list the criteria for the definition of the new disease, as if it were a disease with clear parameters, consisting of unique and specific symptoms, whereas it consists of symptoms that are similar to many other diseases, often occurring at the same time. Hence, we have the terms "lupus-like," "scleroderma-like," and "arthritis-like." This is like asking an oncologist to establish criteria for the diagnosis of lung cancer as if it can be properly classified as lung cancer only if it shares no characteristics with other forms of cancer and is clearly distinguishable from them as a unique disease. This line of defense questioning clearly revealed the legal view of science as providing clear and undisputable fact, whereas scientists acknowledge science as an ongoing, open-ended process of discovery.

Judge McKibben in the *Merlin v. 3M/McGhan* case established that the threshold point was whether Mrs. Merlin had a silicone gel-induced disease or whether she had scleroderma, as if scleroderma or scleroderma-like disease could not be a disease induced by silicone gel breast implants. Dr. Brawer tried to demonstrate that scleroderma was a working diagnosis included as one of the disease compensation categories and did not preclude the umbrella disease of silicone-induced illness. If Dr. Brawer could not convince him that Mrs. Merlin was not just suffering from scleroderma, then the judge indicated that he would have no choice but to "go to the epidemiology," a statement which indicates an assumption that there was no relationship between silicone gel implants and atypical autoimmune disorders.

Daubert might reasonably be expected to expand the information allowable in court, through the determination that if the methodology is appropriate, even if the conclusions are not generally accepted by the medical community, novel studies and findings should be allowed before a jury. However, what seems to be happening is that at least in cases involving breast implants, Agent Orange, and similar products, the manufacturers are attempting to convince judges that "if it isn't epidemiology then it isn't science"; that is, if no epidemiological study supports cause and effect, then there is no relationship.

Judges, as gatekeepers, need to know when epidemiology is the appropriate method and when it isn't; they also need to know when other methods may be more appropriate. While judges and perhaps juries are sometimes convinced that epidemiological studies are good because they study the phenomenon in a large population resulting in definitive findings, in truth, the actual number of people who finally are studied may be very small indeed. For example in the Mayo study, only thirty-two women received the important followup questionnaire and only seventeen of these had implants. Yet the defense purports that this was a long-term national study of thousands of women, providing reliable and valid results. Despite these problems, because certain highly publicized epidemiological studies, defective in their own right, do not show to a 95 percent scientific certainty a significantly increased risk ratio, judges are being asked to conclude that there is no evidence linking silicone gel breast implants with connective tissue disease. The defense hopes that this will translate into a conclusion (actually unwarranted and unrelated to the findings of the epidemiological studies) that breast implants are safe and should be put back on the market. Juries would then not be allowed to conclude that it is more probable than not (i.e., at least 51 percent more likely than not) that a plaintiff's breast implant did cause the woman's disease because the epidemiological studies did not prove this to a 95 percent certainty. Juries would in fact not be allowed to hear cases in which the evidence was under dispute, the very thing that juries are designed to hear and decide. If the justice system is going to become a system in which judges hear the evidence and try it, then what will become of juries? Huber (1991) and Angell (1994), as I state elsewhere, hope that it means that juries disappear from civil cases, especially when the stakes are high and the corporations can buy the evidence.

In *Science on Trial* (1996), Angell presents the breast implant litigation as meaningless until such time as the "truth" about silicone is discovered. In actuality, she is suggesting that we wait for decades, not because there is not danger, but because the peculiarities of this phenomenon cannot be adequately studied now. She suggests implicitly that our tradition of over two hundred years, in which a jury hears both sides of a case and then decides, based on the evidence, be discarded. Yet, the science on which this truth is based is a process of discovery, one open to challenge and dispute on many fronts. If women had to wait for the epidemiology to catch up to their illnesses, it might be decades before they could make a case. A related example is the drug, DES, in which the defense argued successfully for a while that there were no epidemiological studies that showed DES caused uterine cancer in women born to mothers who had taken it. Many women won against the manufacturers in these cases, despite the fact that epidemiological support for a relationship would be a long time coming. When Angell reports that the epidemiological studies do not show any relationship between implants and illness, she is being less than genuine. She is ignoring the cautionary conclusions reached by the researchers, as well as the significant criticisms offered by plaintiffs and consumer groups—primarily that epidemiological studies cannot prove "no causal relationship" just as they do not prove "cause," and second, that the studies on which the defense relies are, from the women's perspective, fatally flawed.

A significant risk facing the plaintiff is that if judges believe that only epidemiology is "real science" and everything else falls short of that (as they seem to in several cases I have reviewed) and if judges don't understand the purposes and limitations of epidemiological studies, then judges may be convinced that if a relationship is not proven using this method, it doesn't exist. Consequently, the plaintiff would have no case. It is, therefore, very important to understand just what epidemiological studies can and cannot tell us. Let us turn first to a description of the purpose and process and limitations of an epidemiological study, and then to the criticisms that are directed against the findings or, more accurately, the way the findings are often reported and used.

Epidemiology in the field of public health studies the "incidence, distribution, and etiology of disease in human populations and applies the findings to alleviate health problems" (Bailey et al., 1994:125). In the courtroom, the findings generated by epidemiological research are often offered to establish or dispute whether exposure to an agent caused a harmful effect or disease. Such has been the case in the legal dispute over whether Bendectin caused birth defects (*DeLuca v. Merrell Dow Pharmaceuticals, Inc.*, 1990), whether swine flu vaccine caused Guillain-Barré disease (*Cook v. United States*, 1982), and whether exposure to Agent Orange and dioxin contaminant caused various illnesses in Vietnam veterans and birth defects in their offspring.

Epidemiological research responds to the question of general causation (could the agent have caused this) rather than specific causation (did the agent cause this in this person). Therefore, these studies are likely to find varying degrees of association between an agent and an illness or disease, and use a measure of relative risk to indicate the strength of association between exposure to an agent and illness. Association is not causation and an association identified may not indicate cause, but a properly designed study allows the researcher to assess the degree of association, or lack thereof, between an agent and an illness. A strong association that is consistently demonstrated in a number of research projects leads a researcher to infer that a causal relationship exists. The lack of a finding of association, however, does not mean that no causal relationship exists. It may mean only that the sample size was not large enough to detect a weak association or that the disease has multiple causes rather than one.

Epidemiological studies are necessarily based on studying large numbers of people, and the measurements of error and risk (which are the hallmark of epidemiological studies) lose their meaning when applied to an individual. The Hill (1965) criteria, which are generally applied to evaluate the possibility of cause and effect in court, acknowledge the complexity of determining the relationship between two phenomena. The strength of association between two things is an important consideration in causation, although a weak association does not rule out a causal relationship. For example, if a tiny minority of the population has the problem in the first place, if it is very rare, then we would not expect to find an increased risk ratio in a large population with the introduction of an agent even if the agent were the cause of the problem. Another caveat is that while consistency of association is important in determining cause, simple consistency should not be taken to imply cause; in fact, cause may be related in an inconsistent manner to effect (Hill, 1965).

While epidemiological studies do not address the question of cause in an individual case, or specific causation, a number of courts in addressing specific causation have grappled with the role played by epidemiological evidence in answering that question. The two issues related to the role of epidemiology in proving individual causation are admissibility *and* sufficiency of evidence to meet the burden of proof (Bailey et al., 1994:166). A rigorous epidemiological study that is methodologically valid should be admissible since it tends to indicate that an issue in dispute is more or less likely.

But a more troublesome issue is the sufficiency of the evidence and the burden of proof. Given that the threshold for the civil burden of proof is "more likely than not," epidemiological studies can be adapted to meet this threshold by adhering to the standard that there is a greater than 50 percent probability that the agent is responsible for the disease. Another alternative is the use of attributable proportion of risk parameter, in which the attributable risk is a measurement of the excess risk that can be attributed to the agent above and beyond the background risk due to other causes. There is additional evidence bearing on causation, such as length of time of exposure, dose of exposure, family history or genetics, and these can be expected to modify any probability based solely on the available epidemiological evidence (Bailey et al., 1994:169). One should remember that scientists can never prove a relationship of cause; rather, they can "reject the null hypothesis, or hypothesis of no relationship" at a certain confidence level. Whether we are in a courtroom or a laboratory, any scientific findings are open to question and should remain so. But the demands of the court are very different from the demands of science.

In *Blum v. Merrell Dow* (1996), Judge Bernstein's opinion is extremely relevant to the way corporations are trying to close the door to the jury by convincing the judge that science reigns: "The objects of investigation, and the purposes of science and a system of justice are very different. Science seeks the discovery of 'universal' principles and their application. A system of justice seeks the just resolution of specific cases and controversies. The goals are different. The approaches are different. The analysis is different" (72). Judge Bernstein's opinion was issued in a Bendectin case, but it could have been written as well in response to the defense's position in the breast implant *Daubert* hearings. He stated that the "testimony revealed a sycophantic relationship between "scientists" and their funding source "Merrell Dow," and he found "circularity of reasoning to prove pre-ordained 'scientific' conclusions, and the use of litigation defense funds for scientific research manipulation" (*Blum v. Merrell Dow*, 1996:70).

In 1992, the FDA decision to effectively remove silicone gel breast implants from the market formally sent a strong message to the public and plastic surgeons (although it is hard to imagine that plastic surgeons weren't well aware of the dangers) about their real and potential danger. Since then, heavy lobbying on the part of the AMA and ASPRS and a powerful public relations campaign have begun to convince plastic surgeons, legislators, and potential jurors that there is no association between silicone implants and illness and disease in implanted women. The extensive media attention given the manufacturer-sponsored epidemiological studies that purportedly showed no correlation between silicone gel breast implants and connective tissue disease promulgated the idea that implants were not dangerous, which may already have had an enormous impact on recent jury trials as well as on potential jurors. Perhaps more importantly, these studies may have shaped the standards by which scientific findings could be introduced to those jurors in the first place. And, beneath all of this, the studies are likely to be communicated to physicians who treat women with implants and who rely on popular media as well as salespersons for the manufacturers.

THE EPIDEMIOLOGICAL STUDIES: LOCAL AND SYSTEMIC PROBLEMS

Amid all the noise about the Harvard (Sanchez-Guerrero et al., 1995) and Mayo (Gabriel et al., 1994) studies, one must remember that, in addition to concern about biases and methodological flaws with these studies, many researchers and many women are far more concerned with local reactions than with systemic reactions. Focus on the local reactions requires that the women and their disfigurement remain visible. Shifting the discussion to thousands of women in Olmsted County or to Harvard nurses removes us from the underlying reality. However, the manufacturers have been fairly successful in shifting the focus of the public and at least a few judges from the injuries suffered by the women to the intricacies and nuances of the scientific method.

Not all epidemiological studies have focused on the systemic problems associated with breast implants. Rather, a number of studies have assessed the local problems that are connected with breast implants. Silverman et al. (1996) completed a thorough review of the epidemiological studies of local and systemic complications attributed to silicone gel breast implants. Relying on epidemiological studies identified on MEDLINE, the authors evaluated the methodology of the studies and their findings. Most of the epidemiological studies have concentrated on the complications resulting in connective tissue disorders and cancer. Studies on the incidence of severe but localized complications such as rupture, capsular contracture, breast pain, disfigurement, and scarring are scarce and often incomplete. In addition to defective design and manufacturing, mammography, closed capsulotomy, age of implant, and trauma or injury to the breast have all been implicated in rupture. However, rupture may be spontaneous or caused by normal wear and tear on the elastomer envelope containing the gel.

The "gold standard" for confirmation of rupture is explanation and inspection of the implant. Some estimates of rupture rates have emerged from studies of women whose implants have ruptured. D. L. de Camara et al. (1989) studied women who sought treatment for symptoms related to their implants. These authors found a relationship between the age of the implant and the condition of the implant at the time of surgery. From 1–9 years, 35.7 percent of the implants had ruptured. After 10–17 years, a full 95.7 percent of the breast implants had ruptured or were leaking. Peters et al. (1994) found that from 2–10 years, 25.6 percent had ruptured, and 53.6 percent had ruptured from 11–26 years and after. Robinson et al. (1995) report that 51 percent of the 495 implant recipients in his study had ruptured implants, and 71 percent had either rupture or severe silicone bleed. The risk of a rupture increased with age of implant, leading Robinson and colleagues (1995) to suggest that women should have them replaced after approximately eight years. Some research also reports the development of silicone granulomas or pseudotumors and the migration of silicone to other parts of the body, including the lymph nodes.

Few studies have followed the rate of capsular contracture, the formation of a capsule around an implant that is a normal part of the expected inflammatory response to any foreign body, even one that is "inert." Contracture results in tightening and hardening of the breast, mild to severe pain, deformity of the breast, or distortion and misplacement of the breast. Asplund's (1996) study reports a 54 percent contracture rate, and other studies reported by Silverman (1996) distinguish between contractures of smooth implants at 58 percent after twelve months and 8 percent for textured (polyurethane foam) ones. Often, these studies are designed to compare different types of implants, and due to different methods and purposes, the range of contracture rate reported in Silverman's (1996) review is estimated to be between 2.5 percent for the textured foam implants and 81 percent for a smooth implant. The recurrence rate of contracture is high, approximating 50 percent according to Burkhardt, as reported in Silverman (1996).

Other problems that have been studied less systematically than connective tissue disease include breast pain, infection, delayed wound healing, hematoma, seratoma, changes in breast or nipple sensation, and galactocele formation. Other negative outcomes include wrinkling, shifting, displacement, extrusion of the implant, or unsatisfactory cosmetic results. While there are frequent reports of these problems, the true incidence rates of these events are unknown. Local reactions are often extremely serious problems. Despite the attention given the epidemiological studies that focus on the relationship between silicone gel breast implants and connective tissue diseases, most of the complaints filed in the bankruptcy case of Dow Corning are based on local complications such as rupture, silicone travel, disfigurement, and distortion (*Mahlum v. Dow Chemical*, 1995).

In the breast implant cases, until the publication of the Harvard and Mayo studies, both sides were citing animal studies and case reports. The defense was now blessed with a period during which the global settlement was being structured and most implanted women were being assessed for placement on the grid. Therefore, not pursuing their cases in court, the defense was able to devote its considerable resources to funding studies that would not only assess the causal relationship between implants and connective tissue diseases, but that, more importantly, would meet the requirements of the new federal standard governing the admissibility of evidence in court: *Daubert*.

The manufacturers were eagerly awaiting the publication of the epidemiological studies in the *New England Journal of Medicine*. These studies, based on large samples, were supposed to help settle the question of the relationship between silicone gel and disease. When they were published, the defense happily cited them as showing no association.

However, a number of authors, including Dr. David Kessler of the FDA in the *Annals of Internal Medicine* (1996), questioned the proffered interpretation that these studies proved no association. While scientists may debate the methods and conclusions of these studies, the defense is rushing forward, waving the findings in the face of judges and jurors. They are asserting that there is now "proof" that breast implants do not cause silicone-related disease.

The best known of the studies assessing the relationship between silicone breast implants and autoimmune and connective tissue disease are those referred to in the press as the Harvard Nurses Study and the Mayo study, but there are others. Silverman and her colleagues, one of whom is David Kessler, review the existing epidemiological research and report the following: Weisman et al. (1988) surveyed 378 patients who had implants. Of the 125 who responded to their questionnaire, none reported any of the diseases of interest to the researchers, including rheumatoid arthritis and systemic lupus. This study was severely flawed by not having a comparison group, unexplained small response rate, and small sample size. Several other studies reported by Silverman (1996) suffer from similar methodological shortcomings, severely limiting the value of their findings. Schusterman and colleagues (1993) prospectively studied patients having breast implants or breast reconstruction, and after a followup of 2.5 and 1.9 years, respectively, found no difference in the incidence of diagnosed rheumatic disease. The fact that all of the patients in the study had breast cancer coupled with the very short follow-up time creates serious problems for this study according to the critique reported in the *Annals of Internal Medicine* (1996). Goldman and colleagues (1995) found that patients with silicone breast implants were no more likely than those without implants to have received a diagnosis of a known (i.e., classic) connective tissue disorder. The fact that the patients were referred patients with a presumed high incidence of rheumatological disorders as well as other methodological problems limits the usefulness of this study.

We turn now to the two most widely cited epidemiological studies. Gabriel and colleagues (1994) conducted a large retrospective cohort study of the association between breast implants and connective tissue disorders among 749 residents of Olmsted County, Minnesota, who received implants between January 1964 and the end of December 1991. They reviewed the medical records of implant recipients and an age-matched comparison group. They found no increased risk of connective tissue disease, cancer, or other problems. This study avoided some of the problems of earlier cited studies but still had a number of problems: it was a records-only study, it was retrospective, and the sample of women with breast implants was very small. Silverman et al. (1996) conclude, however, that despite its flaws, the results of this Mayo study "tend to rule out a marked risk for well-defined connective tissue diseases related to silicone breast implants" (750). This conclusion is not germane to the questions about the relationship between silicone gel breast implants and atypical connective tissue diseases, which are the concern of the women with breast implants.

Sanchez-Guerrero and colleagues (1995) in the Harvard Nurses Health Study conducted a retrospective cohort study of a much larger group— 87,501 women, 876 (or about 1%) of whom had silicone gel implants. These participants had been receiving a biennial questionnaire between 1976 and 1992. On the basis of responses to these questions, the investigators identified a group of participants who had reported a physician's diagnosis of such connective tissue disorders as scleroderma, systemic lupus erythematosus, rheumatoid arthritis, as well as rheumatic or musculoskeletal disease. A total of 5,086 (6 percent of the entire cohort) of the women reported such diseases and were sent a "screening questionnaire" designed to provide more specific information on self-reported signs and symptoms. While this study purports to provide additional evidence against a marked increase in the risk for certain connective diseases or disorders in implant recipients, it does not, because of the sampling process, address whether symptoms of atypical connective tissue disorders occur more frequently in such recipients. This distinction is of great significance in the current litigation because plaintiffs are not claiming an increase in classical connective tissue diseases, but in atypical connective tissue diseases that are similar to recognized, classic diseases. This study, though often cited as proof that silicone gel implants are harmless, clearly speaks to a different issue—whether, in the sample studied, there was a marked increase in the risk of classic connective tissue disease as a result of silicone gel breast implants. One problem with this study is that only those women who reported a defined, physician-diagnosed classic connective tissue disorder were even sent questionnaires. Thus, all of the rest (94 percent of the entire sample of women) were assumed to have no self-reported disorders. This assumption likely led to an underestimation of the prevalence of these symptoms.

Hennekens and colleagues (1996) recently used the Harvard Nurses Study data to study the association between a history of silicone breast implants and self-reported history of connective tissue disease. They actually found a 24 percent increase in the risk of classic connective tissue disease in women with implants, but in their interpretation of the results, they downplayed that increase as "insignificant."

Taken together, these studies suggest no substantial increase in the risk for scleroderma or other well-defined connective tissue diseases as a result of silicone gel breast implants. However, no study has specifically studied *atypical* connective tissue diseases. The few studies that have "glanced at" particular atypical conditions have had serious flaws that have made them inconclusive.

One problem associated with drawing conclusive answers from any of these studies is that the disorders linked to silicone are extremely rare in the general population and are therefore difficult to detect, even in large cohort studies such as the Harvard Nurses Study. For example, as Silverman et al. (1996) point out, the incidence of scleroderma in the general population is between two and ten cases in a million people (751). One can imagine how difficult it is then to develop comparison groups of adequate numbers. In the Mayo Clinic study, the authors found five cases of connective tissue disease among 749 women with breast implants, with ten cases among the 1,498 without implants. This statistic speaks more to the rarity of connective tissue diseases in the population than it does to the relationship between silicone gel and connective tissue disease.

None of the epidemiological studies has concluded that the rate of well-defined connective tissue disease or breast cancer is increased substantially in women with silicone breast implants. However, no study has ruled out a moderately increased risk, and the epidemiologic literature is inadequate to rule out an association between breast implants and connective tissue-like diseases. The authors of the Harvard Nurses Study make no claim that it is a conclusive study: "for this and other reasons, our study cannot be considered definitely negative. . . . The application of strict criteria for any connective tissue disease may exclude some true cases or milder cases and hence underestimate the true incidence of the disease" (Sanchez-Guerrero et al, 1995:1670).

Because of the visibility and significant legal and political importance of the Harvard and Mayo studies, it is important to present the major criticisms of these studies as they relate to the issues relevant in court, both before a judge and eventually before a jury. A number of criticisms of both the Harvard and the Mayo studies cast doubt on the conclusions many manufacturers and their attorneys have drawn from these important studies, primarily related to sample size and selection procedures, case definitions, follow-up, criteria for inclusion of patients, and funding (Silverman et al., 1996).

Let us turn first to the Mayo study. Although the authors reveal that the study was partially funded by the Plastic Surgery Education Foundation (PSEF) of the American Society of Plastic and Reconstructive Surgeons, they do not mention that Dow and other manufacturers gave PSEF money, which was then funneled to Mayo (Noone, 1994). Dow, on the one hand, claims this as a normal research contribution, denying any vested interest in the study or its outcome. On the other hand, Dow claims it as a defense expense in the bankruptcy documents, clearly supporting the plaintiff's claim that Dow was "buying science." Dow admits not only that the purpose of the epidemiological studies was to defend itself, but also that it never intended to produce implants again. Therefore, it was interested in the studies only as evidence to protect itself in court rather than to study possible problems with implants. Initially, then, Dow Corning did not express any interest in the safety of the millions of implants it was producing. Moreover, even when the FDA removed them from the market thirty years later, Dow was still not interested in their safety. It was only interested in its financial health and protecting itself from injured women. James R. Jenkins, Dow Corning's general counsel and vice president, submitted an affidavit in the insurance litigation in which Dow Corning sought reimbursement from Hartford Insurance Company for the money it spent funding the Mayo and Harvard studies. In the affidavit, he states: "In order to defend itself against silicone breast implant claims, Dow Corning funded or contributed funding to a number of internal and external studies which were intended to provide the epidemiological data necessary to defend against allegations of breast implant plaintiffs that their breast implants caused certain diseases" (2). He went on: "Each external scientific study that Dow Corning funded was only after consulting with legal counsel to determine its impact on the breast implant litigation" (*Dow Corning v. Hartford Accident & Indemnity*, 1996:3). Dow admits that these studies, which they tout as totally unbiased, neutral, and methodologically sound, were studies they paid for in order to protect themselves.

Consumer and breast implant support groups are also concerned with both the failure to include atypical connective tissue diseases and the inclusion of nonconnective tissue diseases in the study, which have never been tied to silicone gel implants; ankylosing spondylosis, for example, could not have been expected to vary between the groups they studied. Alarmingly, this totally expected finding is then used by the researchers to support the conclusion of "no increased risk" associated with silicone.

These problems mirror one of the major concerns that plaintiffs have about the impact of the *Daubert* standards: major corporations are paying for and involved in the criticism and construction of the protocols for extensive, expensive studies. They hope these studies will convince the judges in their enhanced gatekeeper roles that the threshold of causation has not been reached, and hence, that the cases against manufacturers should not be heard by a jury. While manufacturers customarily support research on their products, their involvement in the development of the study and interpretation and dissemination of results is extremely troublesome.

Dow Corning and Dow Chemical take the high road in the breast implant litigation in a letter to Judge Sam Pointer who oversees the multidistrict litigation. Their counsel writes: "The ultimate purpose of convening a panel of scientists is to bring *unfiltered scientific principles and process to bear on the litigation*" (Bernick, 1996:2). Yet, other letters and affidavits contradict this assertion. Charles Hennekens, affiliated with Brigham and Women's Hospital of Harvard Medical School (who found, but discounted, an increase in systemic diseases among women with breast implants in his epidemiological study of the Harvard nurses), wrote the following to Ralph Cook of Dow Corning (February 8, 1994), in response to Dow Corning's detailed review of his research proposal: "Thank you for your detailed review of our proposals to examine the potential health effects of breast implants and cosmetic injections. In this letter, we will attempt to address each of the specific issues that you have raised. Under separate cover, Dr. William Terry is responding to your specific budgetary and administrative queries." Cook thanks Dr. Terry for: "Your expressed concerns," "Your excellent suggestions," indicating that "We concur." Nevertheless, Dr. Hennekens maintains that Dow Corning had no "input into the design, conduct, analysis, interpretation, publication, or presentation of the results" (Hennekens et al., 1996).

Clearly, other researchers were concerned about the possible impact of the source of funding. One of these researchers, Dr. Jorge Litvak (1996), writes:

While research funding from private industry is to be commended, in this particular case, financial support was received from Dow Corning, one of the manufacturers of silicone breast implants. This company has been in litigation regularly in the last few years as defendants in the center of the controversy. The lawyers for the company provide, consistently, as their main arguments, data from published articles that seem to favor their position. The statement of the authors of this study that "these data are compatible with prior reports from other cohort studies that exclude a large hazard" will certainly be used again by the lawyers from the company that supported this study in part. (2)

Another difficulty is related to followup. Women were followed to December 31, 1991, or to the date of their last health care visit in Olmsted County, Minnesota, where the Mayo Clinic is located, whichever was earlier. Probably, then, women who had moved or died would not receive questionnaires, nor would they have any subsequent records at the Olmsted clinic to be reviewed. The methodology would have been more accurately portrayed if the authors had indicated that they did no followup of women who left the Mayo health system for any reason and they did not know what happened to them.

The known latency period before developing rheumatological complaints in patients with implants was not appropriately considered. Silicone, like tobacco, has a long incubation period, and one would not expect symptoms for five to seven years. Thus, including women with implants for a short time or excluding those with implants for a long time would affect the results.

Another problem with this and other studies that rely on records is that if the ailment or disorder was not included in the record—that is, if it was not mentioned by the woman or not recorded by her physician—it would not be there. Thus, there could be significant underreporting of the more subtle or less severe symptoms. There also seems to be some slippage between the initial 971 implanted women (149 of whom were excluded for unspecified reasons of not meeting the criteria) and the final 749 reported in the study. Seventy-three women who presumably met the criteria are missing in the analysis (Brautbar, 1996). Related to the issue of bias in research construction and conceptual and operational definitions is the fact that Mayo did not reveal that the Mayo Foundation is and was a defendant in silicone gel breast implant cases at the time of the research.

Perhaps most importantly, due to the restrictions of their criteria for inclusion in the study to definite, diagnosed connective tissue disease, the investigators estimate that they missed almost 80 percent of the patients. Many of these patients may have had atypical rheumatic disease, atypical pulmonary disease, atypical gastrointestinal conditions, and atypical neurological conditions (Brautbar, 1996). Perhaps the main criticism of this study is that it failed to address, or even ask about, atypical presentations of disease. If a woman did not fit the criteria for classic disease, but instead had a constellation of atypical symptoms that were close to but did not fit precisely the classical disease picture, she was treated as a woman who was not sick and she was not counted as sick in the study. As one of Mahlums' attorneys, Geoff White, put it, "The Mayo study was the wrong study, looking for the wrong diseases, which gathered the wrong data from the wrong set of women, which predictably resulted in the wrong conclusions." There are other criticisms, but these are the major ones.

The other study often cited in the press and by defense counsel to prove that implants are safe is the Harvard Nurses Study. First, the reader needs to remember that epidemiological studies do not ask that particular question. Their focus is on the increased risk given a particular agent or element in a group of individuals exposed compared with those not exposed. The Harvard Nurses Study, like Mayo, looked only at the more narrowly defined classical connective tissue diseases. The sample is too small, and the criteria for inclusion are too narrow to catch the potential impact of silicone gel on the implanted women. Only those women who had been diagnosed with definitive connective tissue disease or who had indicated that they had been diagnosed with "other major illness," such as lupus erythematosus, rheumatoid arthritis, and scleroderma, received the followup screening questionnaire. Although one hears a good deal about the thousands of nurses in this study, in fact only thirty-two women actually received the screening questionnaire. Furthermore, the criteria were so narrowly defined that only 1 percent of this middle-aged group of women had "any one of the forty-one signs or symptoms" or laboratory findings seen in connective tissue disease, a percentage Noone (1994) states is less than the 5 percent one could expect in the general population. Despite the fact that the participants would have had to indicate that they had one of the forty-one signs or symptoms, there was no indication of how many nurses had even been asked about or tested for them. Therefore, it is impossible to determine the number who actually had them.

Another significant problem presented by this study is that it included women who had implants for as short a time as thirty days. Although the authors report an average length of implant time of around eight years, averaging in this case is clearly meaningless. One would not expect any connective tissue reactions until five to eight years, or possibly longer. There were other problems such as reporting women who had implants longer than was possible (37.5 and 40.5 years), given that the first implants were not available until 1962. The authors did not adequately explain or justify their assertion that bias resulting from the breast implant controversy required the absolute exclusion of data from women after June 1, 1990.

The problems with implants were not widely known in 1990. It was not until 1992 that there was any significant media coverage of the problems tied to them. And while it is customary for corporations to fund research and while such funding does not necessarily indicate bias or an effort to influence the study or its results, it is possible that a $7 million plus grant to Harvard University's Brigham and Women's Hospital from Dow may have allowed the shaping of questions and their interpretation. This is confirmed by Dr. Graham A. Colditz, co-author of the Harvard Nurses Study, who, although unsure of the exact figure, stated that Dow provided between $5 million and $10 million in funding (Silicone Breast Implants Products Liability Litigation, MDL-926, deposition at 23-24). This is further corroborated by Dr. Matthew H. Laing, also a co-author of the Harvard study (MDL-926, deposition at 49 and at 56). (See also Stauber and Rampton, 1996.) Moreover, Dr. Jorge Sanchez-Guerrero, first author of the Harvard study, gave to Dow Corning in 1992 a draft of the study questionnaire prior to it being sent to the women in the study. This is substantiated by two different documents produced by Dow Corning, one of which is a copy of the questionnaire noting that it was "provided in May 1992 by Dr. Sanchez. This is a supplemental questionnaire that will go out in the next couple of weeks" (Plaintiffs' Steering Committee & Liaison Counsel, MDL-926 Breast Implant Litigation). Laing has also admitted to providing Dow with information about the Harvard study while the study was in progress, although he would not clarify whether Dow had any role in shaping the study methodology (Stauber and Rampton, 1996). Moreover, Dow and other breast implant manufacturers paid consulting fees to authors and reviewers of the Harvard study, including Laing (MDL, deposition at 170-171), Schur (MDL, deposition at 18), and Colditz (MDL, deposition at 90). Laing served as a consultant for the defense with the stipulation that he "didn't want to be an expert's [sic] witness" (MDL, deposition of Matthew Laing, January 21, 1995, Vol. 1 at 235), and Schur agreed to serve as an expert witness for several implant manufacturers (MDL, deposition of Peter Schur, January 21, 1995, Vol. 1 at 19). Colditz also agreed to be listed as an expert for the defense (MDL, deposition of Graham Colditz, January 21, 1995, Vol. 1 at 90).

Silverman et al. (1996) criticize the Harvard study for not including chronic fatigue and fibromyalgia-like syndromes, which have been recognized since 1992 as the most common disorders of women with implants. They indicate that to exclude such common and characteristic disorders from the study violates reasonable methodological and conceptual practice.

Dr. Marc Lappé, expert for the plaintiff, summarized the criticisms in his statement in *Daubert* hearings in the *Merlin v. 3M/McGhan* case (1995) in Reno, Nevada. The epidemiological studies are of limited value because they looked for classic or typical diseases, not atypical connective tissue diseases that are tied to silicone; they did not follow up on the lead of animal studies; and they missed opportunities to study rupture populations and high-risk populations. Lappé specifies that in the Mayo study, only thirty-two questionnaires were finally sent out and only seventeen of those were sent to women with gel implants. The studies were basically designed to find limited information on problems that were actually not the problems one would expect to find related to silicone. In the *Mahlum v. Dow Chemical* case, one of the plaintiff's attorneys (Ellis) summed up the relevance of the Harvard study by drawing a parallel between looking for a relationship between silicone gel implants and classic connective tissue disease and looking for a relationship between cigarette smoking and foot cancer.

While the *Mahlum* trial was in progress in Reno, the American College of Rheumatology (ACR), without a vote from the members, issued a statement that there was no association between silicone gel implants and connective tissue disease. Such a statement was potentially useful to the defense, and the defense had a copy of the board's statement before it was available to the public. Although Judge Steinheimer did not allow the opinion, due to the lack of foundation and the hearsay role it played, it would have been potentially powerful to a jury. The ACR's statement ignored the numerous papers that had been presented at their meeting suggesting a link between silicone gel and atypical connective tissue disease. One cannot ignore the possible implications of the fact that the editors of *Arthritis and Rheumatism*, include Schur and Liang who are also co-authors of the Harvard study and have been listed by the defense as litigation experts. There was no disclosure that they were paid consultants and/or expert witnesses for the manufacturers during the time they published an article entitled "Silicone Breast Implants and Rheumatic Disease: Clinical, Immunologic, and Epidemiologic Studies" (1994) in *Arthritis and Rheumatism*. Their article concluded that the epidemiologic evidence to date did not support the existence of a relationship between breast implants and connective tissue disease. There was no disclosure of the payments breast implant manufacturers made to the authors or to Brigham and Women's Hospital where the study took place. Laing admits that the article submitted to *Arthritis and Rheumatism* doesn't disclose any conflicts (MDL, deposition at 135), nor did he disclose to his colleagues that he was receiving money from the breast implant manufacturers (Colditz MDL deposition at 35 and 41). Colditz also did not disclose to his colleagues that he was receiving money from the breast implant manufacturers while working on the study (Liang MDL deposition at 122-124). Furthermore, the editor of *Arthritis and Rheumatism* invited the president of Dow Corning to submit a "position paper" to that journal (Sheller, 1995). Such an invitation is virtually unheard of for this journal, and the publication committee only discovered it after it was published. It frequently goes unnoticed that in 1996, the American College of Rheumatology, under strong pressure from many of its members, changed its strong statement of "no causation" and instead limited its conclusion to classical diseases. These studies have enormous potential power in court. In the *Merlin* case, Judge McKibben asked why there were no studies challenging the Mayo and Harvard findings. Revealing the difficulty of his position, he inquired as to how the courts were supposed to unravel this problem. Until more study is done, he said, we can't be sure. Therefore, how could one say to a reasonable degree of medical certainty that silicone caused the problem? Judge McKibben expressed the situation he faced in his questions to Dr. Brawer, a plaintiff's witness. At this point, he said to Dr. Brawer, it was premature for Dr. Brawer to draw conclusions from his research and premature to say that epidemiological studies were useful thereby leaving the courts just where they were. (See *Daubert Hearing of Merlin v. 3M/McGhan*, 1993.)

In a nutshell, defense attempts to have the judiciary greatly expand its gatekeeping function could result in the loss of the right to a jury trial by many women with implants. Some pro-manufacturer authors have asserted that the scientific evidence in product liability cases is so complex, and juries so poorly equipped to distinguish scientific fact or empirical data from the courtroom prowess of plaintiff's attorneys, that we should consider abandoning the use of juries in civil cases altogether (Angell, 1996; Huber, 1991). Angell suggests that plaintiffs prefer juries because they tend to give large punitive damages and because they can be manipulated by sophisticated attorneys. Huber (1991) concludes that juries cannot distinguish "junk science" from real science and yet are asked to make multimillion dollar decisions based on scientific evidence. Both of these authors would lean heavily toward limiting the "science" in breast implant cases to the Harvard and Mayo and a few other epidemiological studies, convincing judges that since "no cause" has been proven, the case has no merit. Plaintiffs, of course, rely heavily on clinical studies and shudder at the possibility that a judge may conclude, under *Daubert*, that he or she will "just have to go with the epidemiology," especially if that judge accepts the epidemiology as supported by the defense.

The simple truth is that scientific studies are generally not designed or conducted to serve as good courtroom evidence. When a scientist is called upon to translate the research process with all of its limitations and cautions to the judge and jury, there is a high risk of misunderstanding or confusion not only among the jury, about whom the corporations are so suspicious, but also among the attorneys and judges. However, the attorneys on both sides of the case are expected to bring their scientific theories of causation to the jury by using the 2000-year-old tools of the lawyer's trade—cross-examination, simplification, and summation. In the *Mahlum* case, the jurors became very knowledgeable about the science and history of breast implants after four weeks of very complex testimony in which they developed a clear understanding of the testimony on both sides. Juries can sift through days and weeks of testimony, making clear-headed, thoughtful and well-informed decisions. "The standard of legal proof, a preponderance of the evidence, is not necessarily accepted by science as the proper test, *nor should it be*" (*Blum v. Merrell Dow*, 1996), but it is accepted by the juries.

How reasonable is it to suggest that the jury system be abandoned in civil cases and retained in criminal cases? How would justice be better served in that eventuality? If a jury can't be expected to decide a complex product liability case, is it reasonable to assume it can do any better with a complicated murder case? Suggestions that the jury system be abandoned, when put forward by the corporations and their apologists, are blatantly self-serving. If corporate interests can't push through tort reform to protect themselves, it may be more fitting to cloak themselves in the seemingly neutral mantle of "science" and convince judges to block the jury from its role as decision maker. But "if the law becomes the handmaiden of every self-defining 'science,' each trial judge can delusionally become the arbiter of ultimate reality; and whatever the judge accepts as a 'generally accepted scientific principle' precludes any courtroom challenge" (Bernstein, 1996:46). Therein lies the significant threat of the way the *Daubert* standard is being interpreted today. And as with *Blum v. Merrell Dow* regarding Bendectin, in the breast implant litigation and in all litigation in which "science" is allowed to become the centerpiece, "the testimony . . . about the scientific research and literature on Bendectin should raise a red flag for any judge who considers abdicating the courts' historical role in the resolution of disputes to any scientific establishment" (71).

10

Breast Implants in the Larger Context of Violence Against Women

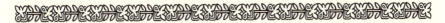

Women are serving as guinea pigs in a vast, uncontrolled clinical trial.

> —Representative Ted Weiss quoted in
> *Tainted Truth* (1994) by Cynthia Crossen

Anne lifted her shirt, unfastened her bra and revealed a chest riddled with scars, concave in places. Smooth, shiny scar tissue covered other areas. There was skin hanging where she once had breasts. She felt maimed. She blamed herself, she blamed her doctor, she blamed Dow Corning. She also thought it was futile to blame. She was sick and she hated her body. She wanted her husband to leave her so she wouldn't feel guilty about not wanting to make love with him. She really wanted to be alone, to disconnect from her painful world. She wanted to die.

Anne typified many of the women we interviewed. She was more damaged and more devastated by what had happened to her body than many, but she illustrates the feeling so many women have of being violated, of being the unknowing victims of silicone. These women are as hard on themselves as they are on anyone else. They are angry, fearful, desperately sad, and hopeless.

After sitting with several of these women and hearing their stories and their feelings about themselves, I was struck by the many similarities between them and victims of rape, sexual harassment, and battery. These forms of violence are brutal, confusing and often devastating. They are the forms of violence that have received the greatest attention from politicians, the women's movement, feminist scholars, social workers, and the media. The resulting analysis and understanding has increasingly focused on the complex structural, cultural, and interpersonal factors in which the violence is embedded. It is this focus that must also be applied to an understanding of breast implants as a form of violence against women. Women who have had breast implants feel assaulted by a chemical that is leaking or bleeding into their bodies, a foreign substance that is knotting or pulling against their skin, causing rashes, fatigue, aches, pain, headaches, memory loss and a pervasive dis-ease. Initially it may seem somewhat extreme to parallel women with implants now suffering various illnesses with victims of battery or sex crimes. But a careful look at the women's medical and social experiences and at others' responses to them reveals undeniable similarities. Rather than approach each of these forms of violence against women as separate and understandable in terms of individual or interactional characteristics unique to the form of violence, we are better served by analysis of the social and cultural context in which they emerge and are constructed as social problems.

First, these forms of violence emerge in a culture characterized and shaped by patriarchy (Dobash, 1979; Steinmetz, Strauss and Gelles, 1980; Estrich, 1987). They are reflected in a social structure characterized by economic and political inequality. Structural and gender inequality reinforce cultural messages as well as the definitions and constructs that are consistent with them. This general connection between violence against women and cultural and structural factors has received a good deal of attention in academic and popular literature and provides us with a framework for understanding the similarities between these more recognized forms of violence against women and breast implants.

One of the most important ties between these types of violence is revealed in the initial definition. At the most general level of analysis, the fact that something is labeled a social problem is the result of either moral entrepreneurs (to use Becker's description of those with a personal stake in a problem) or interest groups, having the power to label it as such and having that label codified and institutionalized. Sexual harassment, rape, marital rape, and battery are all labels effectively applied to behavior after social and legal battles (Gordon, 1988; Conrad and Schneider, 1992). In each of these instances we are clearly dealing not only with behavior, but with definitions and constructions of it, constructions on the part of the individuals involved and the agencies and experts who respond to the event. Sexual intercourse, for example, while a component of most rapes, doesn't alone define it. Rather the expectations, experiences, and definitions of each of the participants shape the event as either intercourse or rape, relying heavily on cultural categories available to both parties.

Similarly, whether a woman is battered or one who gets beaten up now and again is clearly a matter of definition. Both the woman and the experts rely on profiles of batterers and women who are battered or analyses of the interactions between men and women in defining the situation at hand (see Steinmetz et al., 1980; Pagelow, 1989; Loeske and Cahill, 1984). How a situation is defined determines its meaning and the response to it. Women who define being beaten as a customary part of married life are unlikely to define themselves as battered. Shelter workers are committed to translating the woman's experience into a definition of self as "battered woman," one who then can leave the batterer and get help (Loeske and Cahill, 1984). As Gordon points out (1988) women have been beaten for centuries, usually with impunity and often with the expectation that it will be a valuable and necessary lesson. Only recently, and as a result of the women's movement and the grass roots efforts of shelter workers, was such beating redefined as battery. And it is only in the very recent past that battery has been defined as a problem worthy of social or legal intervention. Undeniably, the definitions of this behavior have evolved as a result of interest group activity and have resulted in a legal and political environment that is much different than the one in which the discussion of battery and wife beating first took place.

The power of the definition is apparent in sexual harassment cases. This is particularly clear in the case of "hostile work environment" harassment (MacKinnon, 1979) in which the harassment is a part of the ongoing work place circumstance rather than a request for sexual favors in return for job placement or advancement (*quid pro quo*). In fact, whether a behavior is harassment or not is legally dependent on the woman's definition of reality and her efforts to communicate that to a man (who may have his own definition). Unlike rape, harassment is a legal category of sex discrimination that developed from women's realities and experiences, and as such specifically reflects their definitions of the situation. Nevertheless, women's definitions do not develop in cultural isolation; they are shaped by knowledge and understanding of the implicit rules governing appropriate sexual behavior and gender expectations as well as their response to those rules in particular situations. More specifically, whether the woman's experience is reflective of harassment or battery is a matter of definition and negotiation. She is heavily influenced by the cultural context within which the behavior occurs, and within that context, she must convince herself and others that she is legitimate in her claim that she has been raped, battered, or harassed. This is of course not an entirely straightforward matter. The way the legal system and people in her social network define her experience is a product of her and others' definitions and reactions. An important component of this process of definition is the interpretation of her part in the event, her behavior. The question first posed in each of these instances is usually some form of "what did she do?" This question holds two meanings. First how did the woman precipitate the behavior in question through her actions, dress, location, or demeanor? and second, what was her response to it?—did she submit, retaliate, leave, report it immediately? In all instances, her behavior is as much a part of the definitional process and explanation for the event as is his.

Whether she reported it immediately or waited becomes an important determinant of whether she was a "real victim" from the police and district attorney's point of view (Stewart, 1992). In legal proceedings the woman's behavior is of great significance when determining whether rape, harassment, or battery actually occurred. We are of course most familiar with this in the case of rape, but in battery cases, especially when a woman returns to a battering relationship, and harassment cases, when she has allowed or endured a certain behavior or remark in the past, others frequently look for the part the woman played. The question of responsibility is of paramount importance with breast implantation, just as it is with those other forms of violence against women. In interviews with jurors and discussions with women who have had implants, some of the most common responses were "she did it to herself," "she should have known better," and "it was her own decision—she'll just have to live with the consequences." Jurors as well as general public opinion caution the woman against blaming others and encourage her to accept responsibility for her part in the pain she is experiencing. Those jurors and neighbors and others are correct to a point. She did choose to do it, but she chose implants just as a woman might choose to have coffee with a man who eventually rapes her—in a climate of trust. She could not have predicted the outcome. Blaming a woman in this culture for wanting a more attractive body denies the reality in which women live. Remembering F. Scott Fitzgerald's reference to Zelda as a "fading but still attractive woman of 27" may illuminate the desire of women, especially those between 30 and 50, to do whatever is necessary to remain attractive.

Women who have implants are held responsible for the consequences they suffer, just as are women who are raped or battered. Victims of rape, battery and harassment are frequently rendered ineffective because they feel they were responsible for the crime or assault. They succumb to an incorporation of the cultural definitions of the particular offenses. Their incorporation of definitions of another's reality not only influences the victims' initial decisions after an assault or harassment, but also

shapes their continued reactions. This incorporation of definitions influences whether the women will pursue a charge to its conclusion. When
they do not, recognizing the emotional or financial cost to themselves or
family, they are trapped by cultural explanations that define them as
contributory and untrustworthy or unreliable, hence supporting officials'
claims that pursuing these charges is not worth the effort.

In this regard, Dr. Marcia Angell's (1996) review of the Mariann Hopkins case is eye opening. It reveals her ability to fit almost anything into
the view that the litigation-mad class action attorneys and their clients
are doing their best to destroy corporate America, resulting in the denial
of access to life saving devices for hundreds of thousands of people. The
Hopkins case was attorney Dan Bolton's second major breast implant
case, following *Stern* (Angell, 1996). She had breast implants following a
double mastectomy for fibrocystic disease (as did most of the women
who had mastectomies). The generally accepted practice in the seventies
was to remove fibrocystic breasts so women with a family history of
breast cancer could avoid the risk of cancer. Yet, Marcia Angell (1996)
writes about Mariann Hopkins as if she simply decided on her own to
have a mastectomy and convinced some surgeon that it was necessary
and then pressured him to provide implants. In reality, Hopkins received
implants after a mastectomy she was told to have to prevent cancer. With
the luxury of hindsight unavailable to Mariann Hopkins, or her doctor,
Angell writes:

> Mariann Hopkins of Sebastopol, California, a secretary at Sonoma
> State University in nearby Rohnert Park and the wife of a San Fran-
> cisco firefighter, was in her early thirties when she underwent a
> double mastectomy in 1976 because of fibrocystic disease of the
> breast. This is a very common condition that produces tender nod-
> ules in the breasts, particularly just before menstrual periods.
> Whether it is a precursor of breast cancer or not has been debated
> for decades. The consensus is that it usually isn't, although some
> forms of it may increase the risk. In any case, Hopkins evidently
> did not want to take the chance. (119)

This manner of presentation subtly shifts the focus away from the
known dangers of implants during the seventies and away from the
manufacturers' irresponsibility and fraud. Instead Hopkins is accused of
being overly cautious and willing to go to extremes to avoid the remote
possibility of cancer, even though there was "no agreement" about
whether she was in any danger. This shift to "blame the victim" parallels

asking "what did she do to cause him to rape her?" rather than "why did he rape her?"

As with rape victims or victims of harassment, women who have been damaged by breast implants are not only blamed by others but they readily blame themselves for their disfigurement and illness. They rail against themselves for their stupidity and their vanity. They are ashamed about what has happened; they are ashamed about being sick and about being disfigured. They want to roll back time, turn back the clock, dream it never happened. Some women, sick as they are, with silicone lumps protruding from their collarbones or their breasts, refuse to have them removed, unable to face either the physical or the emotional consequences they anticipate. The parallel with rape victims is stunning. Not only do the victim's friends and families often blame them for being in the wrong place at the wrong time, or dressing or acting inappropriately, so do the police, the district attorneys, and most importantly, so do the victims themselves.

Another important determinant of the definition of the event is an evaluation of how reasonable or understandable or appropriate the woman's behavior was subsequent to the rape, harassment or battery. In fact, her subsequent behavior is incorporated in the definition of the event, and allows for the application of either a label that reflects her experience or one that denies the validity of her claim. For example, whether the woman reported the assault immediately or not is taken by police and district attorneys to be one of the best indicators of whether she was really raped (Stewart et al., 1996). Knowing how police might react to her if she was drinking or invited a man into her house, she may not report it immediately, a factor which then operates against her. In battery cases, her response afterward, especially if she stayed in the relationship or returned to an abusive spouse, affects the definition of her as a legitimate victim. And in cases of sexual harassment, whether she told the harasser that she wasn't comfortable with his behavior or not, and how she responded to him in subsequent interactions has an impact on the definition of the situation as harassment. As with battery or rape or harassment, the legitimacy of a woman's claim that she is sick or damaged as a result of silicone breast implants is derived from her behavior after the event. If she called the police immediately, she is more believable as a rape victim. If she reported the harasser immediately, her claims are more credible. And if she immediately recognized all of her varied symptoms as being related to her implants rather than from working too much, from lupus or some other illness, then her credibility is enhanced. But so often women don't immediately associate their problems with implants and of course neither do their doctors. Even when they do, especially now after so much litigation and a number of well-publicized studies, their doctors may be increasingly likely to discredit the possibility of a causal relationship because the women may not, as in the case of Charlotte Mahlum, go to the doctor often enough, or not make the complaint in a way that leads to it being recorded, or they may not follow the doctor's advice. Unfortunately, the violation women experience in the courtroom is not limited to rape cases. Women's bodies and sexuality make them vulnerable to these attacks in other cases as well. Quite simply, whether the question "what did she do?" refers to her behavior before the event or after it, it reveals an assumption that she may have either precipitated the event, fabricated it, or misinterpreted it. Even the plain-speaking, average American woman, Charlotte Mahlum, was grilled about her relationship with her husband, her sexual maturation, her willingness to seek medical care—anything that could discredit her.

Another area of similarity among rape, harassment, battery, and having breast implants is the inadequacy and ineffectiveness of expert and institutional response. For example, police often discourage a woman from filing a rape charge if her case isn't rock solid, or they doubt the possibility of rape if she knows the accused or has had a sexual relationship with him. They may disparage her if she backs out of her case because of fear, and they may fail to offer her the kind of protection that will make her feel safe (Stewart, Dobbin and Gatowski, 1996). Similarly, women who are abused are sometimes not taken seriously by officials. The attack on them may be redefined as a "domestic dispute" and characterized as reflective of relationship problems rather than as a serious crime. Women who make an effort to pursue harassment charges frequently find themselves outsiders, accused of not being team players, being too sensitive, or lacking a sense of humor (see Dziech and Weiner 1984).

Reliance on experts is expected and encouraged for women who are victims, but they frequently encounter denial, disbelief, or blame. Counselors, for example, may focus on family system problems which they see as characterizing the "dysfunctional family," and they may want to address her "issues of co-dependence" or see her rape as reflective of a mental illness. In each of these instances, some characteristic of the woman makes her culpable. Sometimes the experts' response is to attribute her report of the experience to something unrelated to the experience, suggesting that she was not raped but is merely being jealous, vindictive or attempting to overcome guilt or shame, that she is really just disappointed in the outcome of the relationship, or that she is using her accusation of battery as a weapon to diminish her attacker's claims.

As I point out earlier, in breast implant cases physicians are often unlikely to accept the woman with implants as a legitimate patient. Her
complaints and descriptions are often translated as symptomatic of emotional disturbance or menopause. Furthermore, the medical record constructed through her interaction with her doubting or disbelieving
physician can become an effective weapon in the defense arsenal during
litigation.

Experts in breast implant cases have often responded with disbelief
and rejection of the women who are sick. Their response to women who
want their implants removed reveals their abiding commitment to
women's appearance at all costs. Even when women we interviewed
insisted on removing the implants, some plastic surgeons still refused.
Most simply hand a woman a consent form listing the horrible consequences resulting from removal of the implants. The most commonly
used consent form includes the following check list of complications for
her to acknowledge. This list would dissuade all but the most desperate
women:

- A strong negative impact on my physical appearance, including
  distortion, wrinkling, and significant loss of volume, and/or an
  appearance worse than prior to the initial augmentation.
- Severe psychological disturbance, including depression.
- Loss of interest in sexual relations by either myself or my partner.
- Scar contractures precluding reconstruction later.
- Infection, hematoma (swelling or blood mass), or scarring.
- Loss of breast tissue resulting in loss of breast sensation.
- Inability to breast-feed.
- Implant rupture and inability to remove 100 percent of the resid-
  ual silicone from the breast cavity. (Breast Implant Removal
  Patient Advisory consent form 11.13.97)

The perception of the woman and her understanding of the situation
is often lost, as the police, friends, or attorneys reconstruct the event and
assess the validity of the stories being told. Rather than recognizing the
fluid and emergent definition of the situation, the neighbor, parent, su-
pervisor, or judge inquiring into the woman's role is often measuring
her behavior against a static standard of ideal behavior, which, in hindsight, it seems clear she should have followed. Often, women who attempt to bring charges of rape, harassment, or battery find themselves
in the position of being discounted entirely because they did not conform

to some standard of perfect behavior that could only be determined after the fact. In the breast implant litigation, the women are grilled about when they first noticed symptoms, when they first attributed them to their breast implants. They were expected to have made an immediate connection and pursued it despite the denials and dissuasion by their physicians and even the manufacturers.

The effort to have silicone gel leakage from breast implants accepted as a significant problem is steady and strong, but is countered by assertions that there is no reliable evidence that breast implants cause any problem. Hearings at the FDA and reports to the National Science Panel are contests between manufacturers and plaintiffs, with both vying to have their definition of the situation accepted. The financial, personal and political consequences are substantial. In a similar vein, battery provides an outstanding example of the enormous fight it took to get police, legislatures, and physicians to move violence against women from the status of domestic dispute to felony offense. Still, there is a tendency to treat a man who assaults his wife differently from one who assaults a stranger.

Women who have finally convinced their physicians and attorneys that they are suffering from diseases linked to silicone, or who are being damaged physically by implants, have fought strenuously to have them removed from the market by the FDA. This struggle took decades and is in constant danger (as of this writing) of being reversed. Just when these women were beginning to win some cases in court and to forge asettlement with Dow Corning and other manufacturers, they suffered the devastation of Dow Corning declaring bankruptcy, thereby demolishing the tediously crafted global settlement. The courts and the medical establishment, including practicing physicians and researchers have been unpredictable in their responses to these sick women. A win is often followed by a loss on appeal; a study showing a connection between silicone and sickness is followed by one indicating no association. Physicians' groups such as the ASPRS, the American Medical Association, and the American College of Rheumatology are powerful interest groups intent on convincing both the public and the judiciary that this is a false issue contrived by attorneys and menopausal women.

One of the characteristics most clearly shared by women who have experienced rape, harassment, or battery is the long term impact—the necessity of dealing constructively with a life-altering, self-damaging experience, and building a definition of self that is positive in a climate of disbelief and denial. Therapists build their work around the impact of such experiences on women. They may further victimize women with their definitions, or narrowly reconstruct all of the women's problems as resulting from one particular experience, but they cannot deny the significance of the experiences to the women they see in their practices. The women I interviewed were distressed by the irreversible and avoidable damage they suffered and deeply regretted their irrevocable decision.

CORPORATE DUMPING

The women who have silicone in their bloodstreams are the human counterparts to the rivers of carcinogenic chemicals running through Texas barrios. Their bodies, ravaged by silicone spills reflect the chemical dumps in New York and New Jersey. Not only are women the dumping grounds for corporations with their eyes on the profit margin, they are experimental animals for the manufacturers of silicone gel breast implants, as they were for the Dalkon Shield IUD and DES. This attitude toward women's bodies is not just cavalier; rather, it reflects a deep disregard for women. Just as the land and the fish and animals are destroyed by the strafing and dumping of industry, women's bodies are being systematically devastated by corporate use of them as dumping grounds for dangerous, untested, and potentially fatal, but highly profitable products, here and abroad. If we were talking about one company or one year, we might simply blame an irresponsible CEO or a perverse policy. But we are talking about a process that has been in existence for over thirty years; years during which hundreds of thousands of women have been damaged.

In her book, *Against Our Will* (1975), Susan Brownmiller asserts that during war, women's bodies become men's battlefields. The historically mundane, but personally devastating, act of rape by the victors, illustrates not the effects of testosterone, not just groupthink, but a triumphant signal of dominance to the vanquished through the violation of the women on the losing side. These women lose not just their land, their sons and their husbands, but their bodies and themselves, to the marauding enemy armies. As in gang rape, this is a case of men communicating with one another; women's bodies are simply the turf for the brutal male game of dominance. The fight for access to women's bodies among major chemical and manufacturing companies is no less real; neither are the devastating consequences.

While less immediately and obviously devastating, bodies into which silicone has spilled are the ruins of the war women fight with themselves; the war against aging, against uselessness, against loss. These bodies are battlefields in the war that cannot be won, the fight for everlasting youth and beauty and, ultimately, self-worth. And while the most obvious and immediate attacks are on the self, they are ultimately carrying out the orders handed down in the culture wars. Their bodies are the conduits through which men communicate with other men, illustrating their success or dominance or worth. Women's bodies are advertisements of conspicuous consumption, display cases through which men can demonstrate and find their value. Women are valuable as long as they are useful in this way, and knowing that, women go to enormously expensive, painful and outrageous lengths to "keep themselves up," not "let themselves go" so that men in turn will keep them or not let them go.

The debate about silicone gel breast implants continues. On November 21, 1997, Dow Corning's plan for reorganization under Chapter 11 bankruptcy was denied by Judge Spector. He ruled that, among other problems, the plan provides for an unlawfully coercive voting mechanism, contained improper release provisions, permitted Dow Corning to maintain improper control over the Litigation Trust, and treated foreign claimants unfairly. In October 1997, the FDA again determined that it did not have sufficient information to change the current regulatory policy on silicone gel breast implants, thereby keeping them off the market except in the controlled cases that are ongoing. Five years after the FDA requested safety and effectiveness data from the manufacturers, they had still not provided data adequate to allow the FDA to approve or deny premarket approval (PMA) applications for silicone gel-filled implants. In September, the National Cancer Institute, to much misguided fanfare by the manufacturers and their lobbyists, concluded what the plaintiffs had always known; there was no link between silicone breast implants and breast cancer, but the possibility was serious enough to require continuing study.

Books and articles continue to either proclaim the inadequacy of the jury system when addressing multimillion dollar civil cases or claim the safety of silicone gel breast implants. Marcia Angell's book resulted in a significant display of legitimacy for the manufacturers of silicone gel breast implants. She subsequently appeared on a number of news programs and has become the corporate spokesperson for the position that implants are safe. In November 1997, she received the prestigious William Harvey Award and the Eric Martin Award for medical writing for her book *Science on Trial*, which are sponsored by the American Medical Writers Association, the National Heart, Lung and Blood Institute, and not surprisingly, Bristol-Myers Squibb Co., a breast implant manufacturer. The litigation continues; a consortium of eleven national law firms filed a class action lawsuit against Dow Chemical Company in the United States District Court for the Eastern District of Michigan on Tuesday, October 14, 1997. This follows on the heels of an August decision in a class action suit that found that Dow Chemical did research and testing of silicone for human implantation on behalf of Dow Corning (the same finding as in the *Mahlum v. Dow Chemical* case in Nevada in 1995). Such verdicts for the plaintiffs have been the impetus for Dow Chemical, which had claimed absolute separateness from Dow Corning in *Mahlum*, to consolidate breast implant claims against Dow Chemical and Dow Corning.

At present some 10,000 silicone breast implant cases against the two companies are consolidated in the Eastern District of Michigan before Federal Judge Denise Paige Hood, as ordered by the 6th Circuit (Van Voris, November 24, 1997). The litigation and settlements continue as do disputes about the long term safety of silicone gel-filled breast implants.

The argument to keep breast implants available to women is sometimes deceptively structured around issues of freedom of choice, framed as a feminist or women's rights issue. Such was the claim recently by Anna Vondrak, a Washington-based journalist who frequently writes about women's health issues. She concludes that the FDA's refusal to reinstate silicone gel breast implants resulted from the vociferous opposition by several hundred trial lawyers who were heavy contributors to President Clinton and the Democratic National Committee (Keithley-Johnston, October 23, 1997). Vondrak's claim ignores the reality that many of those lobbying for the availability of silicone gel-filled breast implants are members of groups with corporate financial support.

The claim, also asserted by Vondrak, that implants serve an important need for women and that their availability is a feminist issue is clearly disingenuous. The women clamoring for these rights support few other rights for women. But framing the discourse in this manner appeals to the American values of individual determination and individual rights. When Barbara Vucanovich, former Representative from Nevada, presented her efforts to keep implants on the market as a fight for women's right to independence and freedom of decision-making, she simultaneously fought against family leave, welfare rights, affirmative action, abortion, and every other effort to free women and to improve their lives. One suspects that the concern may be more about keeping manufacturer's profit margins high than about women's right to have implants.

The story about silicone gel breast implants is about women, just as are the stories of harassment, rape and battery. But this story is also about major corporations and business interests engaging in chemical assaults on women. Although the effects of silicone spills in women's bodies may not be immediately obvious, the effects can be worse than the most severe beating. The humiliation and loss of self can be greater than that experienced in harassment, and the feelings of violation, together with the depression and self-hatred, can be as great as in the case of rape.

The discrepancy between the presentation of implants as a beauty aid and the reality of them as physical, financial, and emotional devastation cannot be overstated. There is no way to make this story have a happy ending. Many of the women only want to live long enough to see Dow Corning and other companies pay. Many of them will continue living in pain for the rest of their lives; they have seen their strength fade and their relationships deteriorate. The only bright spot is the plaintiff attorneys' continuing success in their fight against the corporations. This fight is waged not only against manufacturers, but against all the special interest groups who are lobbying for a limit on punitive damages under the rubric of tort reform, and who are lobbying to destroy the jury system through veiled efforts to convince judges that these cases should never go to court. Corporate interests attempt to shape the training judges receive about the admissibility of evidence; they produce epidemiological studies and construct media campaigns to convince women, their families, judges and potential jurors that breast implants are safe. The truth is that for many women, breast implants are toxic, resulting in severe local complications, insidious diseases, and the eventual destruction of their bodies and their lives.

The parallels between the damage caused by breast implants and that caused by the Dalkon Shield IUD are chilling. Of the estimated 110,000 women who conceived despite having the Dalkon Shield, approximately 66,000 miscarried and tens of thousands suffered septic spontaneous abortions. Hundreds of women gave birth to stillborn babies or babies with serious birth defects including cerebral palsy, blindness, and mental retardation. Women who were left infertile received minimal compensation. The average payment was only $2,000 (Robbins, 1996).

In the Dalkon Shield case, Judge Miles Lord, U.S. District Judge for Minnesota, on February 29, 1984 made the following statement to three officers of the A.H. Robbins Company, the manufacturer of the Dalkon Shield. His statement could just as easily apply to the defendants in the breast implant litigation.

> These litigations must be viewed as a whole. Were these women to be gathered together with their injuries in one location, this would be denominated a disaster of the highest magnitude. . . . If one poor young man were, by some act of his—without authority or consent—to inflict such damage upon one woman, he would be jailed for a good portion of the rest of his life. And yet your company, without warning women, invaded their bodies by the millions and caused them injuries by the thousands. And when the time came

for these women to make their claims against your company, you attacked their characters . . . You exposed these women—and ruined families and reputations and careers in order to intimidate those who would raise their voices against you. You introduced issues that had no relationship whatsoever to the fact you planted in the bodies of these women instruments of death, or mutilation, or disease. (Robbins, 1996)

And so it is for women with silicone gel-filled breast implants. But it is also true that the women and their attorneys and the researchers who are convinced of the manufacturers' responsibility for their illnesses and their disfigurement will be in courtrooms across this country until the corporations have compensated the victims for what Judge Lord labels "corporate irresponsibility at its meanest."

APPENDIX

Evidence Photographs

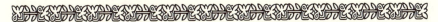

The woman in the photographs had implants following a bilateral sub-cutaneous mastectomy for severe fibrocystic disease.

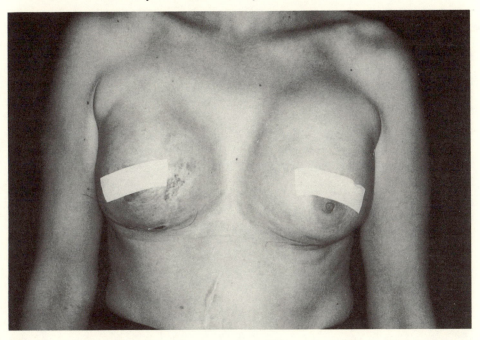

Implant placed through mammary crease, nipple moved, infection with separation of incision and necrosis of central area (August 1978).

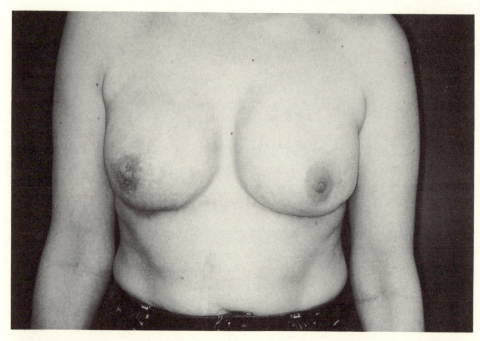

Post-implant, misshapen left implant, right nipple partially removed (March 1979).

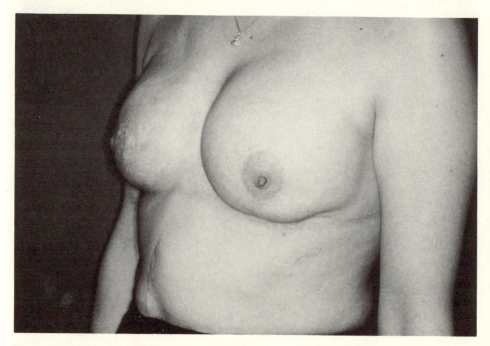

Eleven months post-implant, scarring and dimpling of right implant, swelling and "pocketing" of left, rupture of right (July 1979).

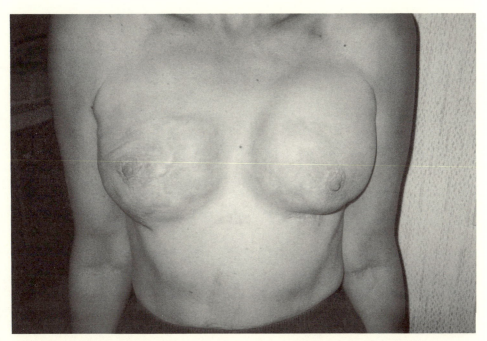

Immediate pre-explant, deformity of both breasts, contracture, rupture (August 1993).

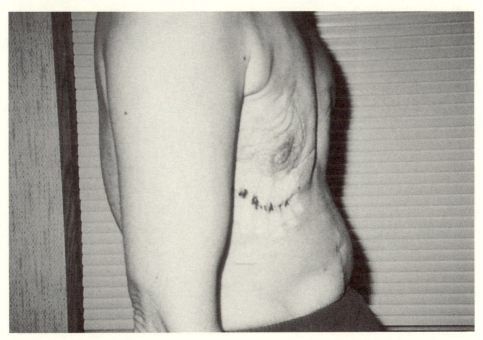

Immediate post-explant (August 1993).

Glossary

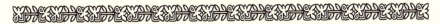

Atypical connective tissue disease A form of disease symptomized by dry eyes, dry mouth, arthritis, and various symptoms similar to arthritis and neurological damage.

Autoimmune diseases Chronic, often deadly diseases, in which there is an apparent immunological reaction of the body against its own tissues; these diseases include rheumatoid arthritis, multiple sclerosis, and lupus erythematosus. They are classified into organ-specific (against one organ, i.e., Addison's disease) and nonorgan-specific (lupus erythematosus) disease.

Capsular contracture Scar tissue formed around the implant. An inflammatory reaction; can cause breast distortion and painful hardening of the breast.

Closed capsulotomy Forcefully squeezing the breast by hand to rupture the scar tissue; also ruptures the envelope causing sudden release of silicone gel.

Connective tissue disease A group of disorders that includes rheumatoid arthritis, systemic lupus, Sjögren's syndrome, dermatomyositis, systemic sclerosis, and other related disorders.

Elastomer The solid silicone material from which the envelope is made.

Encapsulation Enclosure in a sheath not normal to the part, or the process of formation of a capsule or sheath about a structure.

Esophageal immotility The inability of the esophagus to function.

Fibrocystic breast Single or multiple lumps in the breast; the cysts are often harmless and fairly common, but they may be cancerous.

Fibromyalgia Chronic pain in muscles and soft tissues surrounding the joints; reflects a history of widespread pain in one part of the body.

Gel bleed A situation that occurs because the silicone envelope is semi-permeable and substances pass through it in either direction without a rupture of the envelope (elastomer).

Gel migration The tendency for silicone gel to travel to parts of the body outside the breast elastomer.

Global settlement An agreement between the parties in breast implant litigation in which the settling defendants agreed to pay $4,225,070,000, the largest amount ever in a products liability suit.

Human adjuvant disease Defined by the presence of six conditions, including autoimmune disease-like symptoms and signs that develop in patients after plastic surgery involving injections of foreign substances.

Inert Not reacting with other elements.

Inflammation A nonspecific immune response that occurs in response to any type of bodily injury. Reactions may be harmful, including hypersensitivity reaction; processes that lead to rheumatoid arthritis could develop, or excessive scar formation can result.

Lupus erythematosus An autoimmune disorder in which the body's immune system attacks the connective tissue. Sufferers experience malaise, fever, lost appetite, nausea, joint pain, and weight loss, among other symptoms.

Macrophage(s) Any large cell that can surround and digest foreign substances in the body, as protozoa or bacteria; found in liver, spleen, and connective tissue.

Mastectomy Surgical removal of the breast.

Polyurethane Any of various thermoplastic or thermosetting resins, widely varying in flexibility, used in tough chemical-resistant coatings and in adhesive forms, and in electrical insulation.

Raynaud's disease Form of arthritis associated with painful swelling of the fingertips and bluish or white color changes of the hands, especially upon exposure to cold.

Rupture Condition that occurs when the silicone elastomer envelope is breached, allowing gel to escape. Rupture can be caused by capsular contracture, manufacturing defects, daily stresses, stresses during implantation, or external trauma.

Scleroderma A fibrotic thickening characterized by excessive deposits of collagen and other connective tissue in the skin and internal organs and joints. It is characterized by swallowing difficulty, shortness of breath, high blood pressure, joint pain, stiffness, and muscle weakness. It can lead to death.

Silica Crystalline compound occurring as quartz, sand, flint, and other minerals, used to manufacture concrete and glass.

Silicone Any of a group of polymers used in adhesives, lubricants, paints and protective coatings, synthetic rubber, and prosthetic body parts. Silicone gel (as in implants) is a thick, nonsolid form.

Sjögren's syndrome A form of arthritis, characterized by dry and scaly skin, mental deficiency, spastic paralysis, dry eyes, dry mouth, and swollen lymph glands.

Subcutaneous mastectomy Surgery in which all breast tissue is removed, leaving the skin, areola, and nipple intact. Lymph nodes and muscles are not removed.

TDA Chemical 2, 4-tolvenediamine; causes cancer in rats and is suspected of being a human carcinogen.

Bibliography

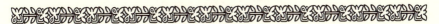

American Psychiatric Association. 1994. *Diagnostic and Statistical Manual of Mental Disorders*. Washington, D.C.: APA.

American Society of Plastic and Reconstructive Surgeons. 1982. *ASPRS Petition to the FDA on Proposed Classification of Inflatable Breast Prosthesis and Silicone Gel-Filled Breast Prosthesis*. Chicago: ASPRS

American Society of Plastic and Reconstructive Surgeons. 1990. *Straight Talk about Breast Implants*. Arlington Heights, Ill.: ASPRS.

Anderson, Margaret. 1996. *Thinking about Women: Sociological Perspectives on Sex and Gender*. Boston: Allyn and Bacon.

Andrews, J. M. 1996. "Cellular behavior to injected silicone fluid: A preliminary report." *Plastic and Reconstructive Surgery* 38:581–583.

Angell, Marcia. 1992. "Breast implants—Protection or paternalism?" *New England Journal of Medicine* 326:1695–1696.

Angell, Marcia. 1994. "Do breast implants cause systemic disease? Science in the courtroom." *New England Journal of Medicine* 24:1748.

Angell, Marcia. 1996. *Science on Trial: The Clash of Medical Evidence and the Law in the Breast Implant Case*. New York: W.W. Norton.

Annals of Plastic Surgery. 1983, November, vol. II. Boston: Little, Brown. (Dow Corning Wright advertisement. "What were you doing in '62?").

Argenta, Louis C. 1983. "Migration of silicone gel into breast parenchyma following mammary prosthesis rupture." *Aesthetic Plastic Surgery* 7:253–254.

Asplund, O., L. Gylbert, G. Jurell, and C. Ward. 1996. "Textured or smooth implants for submuscular breast augmentation: A controlled study." *Plastic and Reconstructive Surgery* 97:1200–1206.

Bailey, Linda, L. Gordis, and M. Green. 1994. "Reference guide on epidemiology." *Reference Manual on Scientific Evidence*. Federal Judicial Center.

Barker-Benfield, G. J. 1976. *The Horrors of the Half-Known Life*. New York: Harper and Row.

Beale, S., G. Hambert, H. O. Lisper, et al. 1984. "Augmentation mammoplasty:

The surgical and psychological effects of the operation and prediction of the result." *Annals of Plastic Surgery* 13:279–297.

Beattie, M. 1987. *Co-dependent No More*. New York: Harper/Hazelden.

Beauty and the Breast: Silicone Implants: A Ms. special report on the ongoing cover-up and continuing controversy. 1996, March/April. *Ms*. pp. 45–63.

Becker, Howard S. 1963. *Outsiders: Studies in the Sociology of Deviance*. New York: Free Press.

Bem, S. 1983. "Gender schema theory and its implications for child development: Raising gender aschematic children in a gender-schematic society." *Signs* 8:598–616.

Ben-Hur, N., and Z. Neuman. 1965. "Siliconoma—another cutaneous response to dimethylpoly-siloxane." *Plastic and Reconstructive Surgery* 36:629–631.

Berger, P. 1963. *Invitation to Sociology: A Humanistic Perspective*. Garden City, N.Y.: Doubleday.

Berger, Peter, and Thomas Luckmann. 1967. *The Social Construction of Reality*. Garden City, New York: Anchor-Doubleday.

Bernick, David. 1996, July 10. Letter to Judge Sam Pointer.

Berscheid, E., E. Walster, and G. Bohrnstedt. 1973. "The happy American body: A survey report." *Psychology Today* 7:119–131.

Best, R. 1983. *We've All Got Scars*. Bloomington: Indiana University Press.

Biggs, T. M., J. Cukier, and L. E. Worthing. 1982. "Augmentation mammoplasty: A review of 18 years." *Plastic and Reconstructive Surgery* 69:449.

Birtchnell, S., P. Whitfield, and J. H. Lacey. 1990. "Motivational factors in women requesting augmentation and reconstruction mammoplasty." *Journal of Psychosomatic Research* 34:509–514.

Blum v. Merrell Dow. 1996, December 13, Court of Common Pleas of Philadelphia County, 1027.

Boot, M. 1996, June 19. "King John's guide to breast implant riches." *The Wall Street Journal*, p. 21.

Bordo, S. 1989. "The body and the reproduction of femininity: A feminist appropriation of Foucault." *Gender/Body/Knowledge*. New Brunswick, N.J.: Rutgers University Press.

Bordo, S. 1993. *Unbearable Weight: Feminism, Western Culture, and the Body*. Berkeley: University of California Press.

Branch, Margaret. "Guinea pigs again: Women's rights in health issues, plastic surgery, breast implants, and other procedures." *Women Trial Lawyers Caucus Newsletter*, 2–5.

Brautbar, N. 1996. "Critical analysis of the most recent New England study claiming no association between silicone breast implants and connective tissue disease." Unpublished.

Brautbar, N., A. Campbell, and A. Vojdani. 1995. "Silicone breast implants and autoimmunity: Causation, association, or myth?" *Journal of Biomaterial Science—Polymer Edition*, 7(2):133–145.

Breast implant litigation settlement agreement: Silicone-gel breast implant products liability litigation. 1993. MDL 926. CV-92-P-10000-S.

Breast Implant Removal Patient Advisory Consent Form. 1997, November 13.

Bridges, A., and F. Vasey. 1993. "Silicone breast implants: History, safety, and potential complications." *Archives of Internal Medicine* 153:2638–2644.

Brinton, L. A., K. E. Malone, R. J. Coates, J. B. Schoenberg, C. A. Swanson, J. R. Daling, and J. L. Stanford. 1996. "Breast enlargement and reduction: Results from a breast cancer case-control study." *Plastic and Reconstructive Surgery* 97:269–275.

Brown, S. L., B. G. Silverman, and W. A. Berg. 1997. "Rupture of silicone-gel breast implants: Causes, sequelae, and diagnosis." *The Lancet.* 350(9090): 1531–1537.

Brownmiller, Susan. 1975. *Against Our Will.* New York: Simon and Schuster.

Brownmiller, Susan. 1984. *Femininity.* New York: Fawcett Columbia.

Brozena, S. J., N. A. Fenske, C. W. Cruse, C. G. Espinoza, F. B. Vasey, B. F. Germain, and L. R. Espinoza. 1988. "Human adjuvant disease following augmentation mammoplasty." *Archives of Dermatology* 124:1383–1386.

Burton, Thomas M. 1996, February 28. "Breast-Implant Study Is Fresh Fuel for Debate." *The Wall Street Journal,* p. B1.

Byrne, John A. 1996a, March/April. "How silicone ended up in women's breasts." *Ms.,* pp. 46–50.

Byrne, John A. 1996b. *Informed Consent: Inside the Silicone Breast Implant Crisis.* New York: McGraw-Hill.

Callaghan, Karen A., ed. 1994. *Ideals of Feminine Beauty; Philosophical, Social, and Cultural Dimensions.* Westport, Conn.: Greenwood Press.

Cermack, T. L. 1986. "Diagnostic criteria for codependency." *Journal of Psychoactive Drugs,* Jan.–Mar. 18(1):15–20.

Chapkis, W. 1986. *Beauty Secrets: Women and the Politics of Appearance.* Boston: South End Press.

Chenoweth, M. B. 1956. "The physiological assimilation of Dow Corning 200 fluid." Internal document.

Chestney, P. L. 1994. "Silicone Victims." Unpublished manuscript.

Chisholm, Patricia. 1992, March 9. "Anatomy of a nightmare." *Maclean's,* pp. 42–43.

Cocke, W. M. 1978. "Nutcracker technique for compressing rupture of capsules around breast implants." *Plastic and Reconstructive Surgery* 62:722.

Cohen, I. Kelman. 1994. "Guest editorial: Impact of the FDA ban on silicone breast implants." *Journal of Surgical Oncology* 56:1.

Cook v. United States, 545 F. Supp. 306:307–316. N.D. Cal. 1982.

Cooley, C. H., 1902. *Human Nature and the Social Order.* New York: Scribner's.

Conrad, Peter. 1992. "Medicalization and social control." *Annual Review of Sociology* 18:209–232.

Conrad, P., and J. Schneider. 1992. *Deviance and Medicalization: From Badness to Sickness*: Philadelphia: Temple University Press.

Cowitiss, E. H., R. M. Goldwyn, and G. W. Anastazi. 1979. "The fate of breast implants on the infections around them." *Plastic and Reconstructive Surgery* 63:812.

Cronin, T. D., and J. Gerow. 1964. "Augmentation mammoplasty: A new 'natural feel' prosthesis." *Transactions of the Third International Congress of Plastic Surgery.* Amsterdam: Excerpta Medica Foundation. 41–49.

Crossen, Cynthia. 1994. *Tainted Truth: The Manipulation of Fact in America*. New York: Simon and Schuster.

Cuellar, M. L., O. Gluck, J. F. Molina, C. Gutierrez, C. Garcia, and R. Espinoza. 1995. "Silicone breast implant-associated musculoskeletal manifestations." *Clinical Rheumatology* 146:667–672.

Cutting, W. C. 1952. "Toxicity of silicones." *Stanford Medical Bulletin* 10(1): 23–26 (Record no. 0789.)

Daly, Mary. 1978. *Gyn/Ecology*. Boston: Beacon Press.

Daubert v. Merrell Dow Pharmaceuticals, 92–102, 113 S.Ct. 2768 1993.

Davis, K. 1991. "Remaking the she-devil: A critical look at feminist approaches to beauty." *Hypatia* 6:21–43.

Daw, J. L., V. L. Lewis, and J. W. Smith. 1996. "Chronic expanding hematoma within a periprosthetic breast capsule." *The Journal of Plastic and Reconstructive Surgery*, 1469–1471. vol 97.

de Beauvoir, S. 1952. *The Second Sex*. New York: Bantam Books/Alfred A. Knopf.

de Camara, D. L., J. M. Sheridan, and B. A. Kammer. 1993. "Rupture and aging of silicone gel breast implants." *Plastic and Reconstructive Surgery* 91:828–834.

Delage, C., J. J. Shane, and F. B. Johnson. 1973. "Mammary silicone granuloma: Migration of silicone fluid to abdominal wall and inguinal region." *Archives of Dermatology* 108:104–107.

DeLuca v. Merrell Dow Pharmaceuticals, Inc. 911 F. 2nd. 941:945–948, 953–959, 3rd Circuit, 1990.

Deutsch, F. M., C. M. Zalenski, and M. E. Clark. 1986. "Is there a double standard for aging?" *Journal of Applied Social Psychology* 16:771–785.

Dobash, R. E., and R. P. Dobash. 1979. *Violence Against Wives*. New York: Free Press.

Dobash, R. E., and R. P. Dobash, 1992. *Women, Violence and Social Change*. London: Routledge.

Dodd, F. J., H. A. Donegan, W. G. Kernohan, R. V. Geary, and A. B. Mollan. 1993. "Consensus in medical communication." *Social Science and Medicine* 37:565–569.

Dow Corning v. Hartford Accident and Indemnity. Case #93–325788CK. Affidavitt of James R. Jenkins.

Dow Corning Corp. v. Hopkins, 115S. Ct. 734 (1998).

Dull, D., and C. West. 1991. "Accounting for cosmetic surgery: The accomplishment of gender." *Social Problems* 38:54–70.

Dworkin, Andrea. 1974. *Woman Hating*. New York: E. P. Dutton.

Dziech, B. W., and L. Weiner. 1984. *The Lecherous Professor: Sexual Harassment on Campus*. Boston: Beacon Press.

Edgley, C., and D. Brissett. 1990. "Health Nazis and the cult of the perfect body." *Symbolic Interaction* 13:257–279.

Ehrenreich, B., and D. English. 1978. *For Her Own Good*. Garden City, N.Y.: Anchor-Doubleday.

Ehrenreich, B., and D. English. 1986. "The sexual politics of sickness." In P. Conrad and R. Kerns, eds., *The Sociology of Health and Illness*, pp. 281–296. New York: St. Martin's Press.

Ellenbogen, R., and L. Rubin. 1975. "Injectable fluid silicone therapy." *Journal of the American Medical Association* 234:308–309.

Epstein, S. 1994, September 9. "Perspective on implants: Women at risk are still in the dark." *Los Angeles Times.*

Erikson, E. 1968. *Identity: Youth and Crisis.* New York: W. W. Norton.

Estrich, S. 1987. *Real Rape.* Boston: Harvard University Press.

Evans, G. R. D., D. T. Netscher, M. A. Schusterman, S. S. Kroll, G. L. Robb, G. P. Reece, and M. J. Miller. 1995. "Silicone tissue assays: A comparison of nonaugmented cadaveric and augmented patient levels." *Plastic and Reconstructive Surgery* 97:1207–1214.

Face to Face with Connie Chung, December 10, 1990.

F.A.I.R. Fairness & Accuracy in Reporting. 1996, January/February, 9:1.

Faludi, Susan. 1992. *Backlash: The Undeclared War Against American Women.* New York: Crown.

Fausto-Sterling, A. 1985. *Myths of Gender.* New York: McGraw-Hill.

Fee-Fulkerson, K., M. R. Conway, E. P. Winer, C. C. Fulkerson, B. K. Rimer, and G. Georgiade. 1996. "Factors contributing to patient satisfaction with breast reconstruction using silicone gel implants." *Plastic and Reconstructive Surgery* 97:1420–1425.

Fertig, Jan. 1993. "Body Image in Adoptees." Unpublished manuscript.

Findlay, Steven. 1992, March 2. "New limits, more questions: Making sense of the latest headlines in the breast-implant controversy." *U.S. News & World Report,* p. 61.

Finkelstein, J. 1991. *The Fashioned Self.* Cambridge, Mass.: Polity Press.

Fisher, J. 1992. "The silicone controversy: When will science prevail?" *New England Journal of Medicine* 326:1696–1698.

Flick, J. A. 1994. "Silicone implants and esophageal dysmotility: Are breast-fed infants at risk?" *Journal of the American Medical Association* 271:240.

Foucault, M. 1973. *The Birth of the Clinic: An Archeology of Medical Perception.* New York: Pantheon.

Foucault, M. 1977. *Discipline and Punishment.* New York: Pantheon.

Franzoi, S. L., J. J. Kessenich, and P. A. Sugrue. 1989. "Gender differences in the experience of body awareness: An experiential sampling study." *Sex Roles* 21:449–515.

Freedman, Rita. 1986. *Beauty Bound.* Lexington, Mass.: D. C. Heath and Co.

Friedson, E. 1970. *Profession of Medicine.* New York: Dodd, Mead and Co.

Frye v. United States, 293 F 1013 D. C. Cir., 1923.

Gabriel, S., W. M. O'Fallon, L. Kurland, M. Beard, J. Woods, and J. Melton, 1994. "Risk of connective-tissue diseases and other disorders after breast implantation." *New England Journal of Medicine.* 330(24):1697–1702.

Gelles, R. G. 1980. "Violence in the family: A review of research in the seventies." *Journal of Marriage and the Family* 42(4):873–885.

Gerlach, Lee, and V. Hine. 1970. *People, Power and Change: Movements of Social Transformation.* Indianapolis, Ind.: Bobbs-Merrill.

Getz, J. A., and H. K. Klein, 1994. "The frosting of the American woman: Self-esteem construction and social control in the hair salon." In K. Callaghan, ed., *Ideals of Feminine Beauty.* Westport, Conn.: Greenwood Press.

Giaretto, H. 1980. *Humanistic Treatment of Father/Daughter Incest: Sexual Abuse of Children*. DHDD Publication No. ADM 78–30161. Washington, D.C.: U.S. Government Printing Office.

Gilthay, E. J., H. J. B. Moens, A. H. Riley, and R. G. Tan, 1994. "Silicone breast prosthesis and rheumatic symptoms: A retrospective follow up study." *Annals of Rheumatic Diseases* 53:194–196.

Global settlement proposal published. 1993. *Mealey's litigation reports: Breast implants*. 1 (21a). Wayne, Pa.: Mealey's Publications. #18–930917–101.

Goffman, E. 1963. *Stigma*. Englewood Cliffs, N.J.: Prentice-Hall.

Goffman, E. 1976. *Gender Advertisements*. New York: Harper Colophon.

Goin, M. K., and J. M. Goin, 1981. "Midlife reactions to mastectomy and subsequent breast reconstruction." *Archives of General Psychiatry* 38:225–227.

Goldman, J. A., J. Greenblatt, R. Joines, L. White, B. Alyward, and S. H. Lamm. 1995. "Breast implants, rheumatoid arthritis and connective tissue disease in a clinical practice." *Journal of Clinical Epidemiology* 48:571–582.

Gordon, L. 1988. *Heroes of Their Own Lives: The Politics and History of Family Violence, Boston 1880–1960*. New York: Penguin Books/Viking.

Gordon, Suzanne. 1991. *Prisoners of Men's Dreams*. Boston: Little, Brown and Co.

Graham. J. A., and A. J. Jouhar. 1983. "The importance of cosmetics in the psychology of appearance." *International Journal of Dermatology* 22:153–156.

Greenlick, M. 1996. "Appendix to Judge Robert Jones' opinion in *Hall v. Baxter Health Care Corp.*" *947 F supp. 1387*.

Grunert, B. K., D. L. Larson, and R. C. Anderson. 1994. "What influences public perceptions of silicone breast implants?" *Plastic and Reconstructive Surgery* 94:318.

Hall v. Baxter Healthcare Corp., 947 F Supp. 1387 (Oregon, 1996).

Handel, N., D. Wellisch, and M. J. Silverstein. 1993. "Knowledge, concern, and satisfaction among augmentation mammoplasty patients, with invited discussion by Garry S. Brody, MD." *Annals of Plastic Surgery* 30:13.

Hatcher, C., L. Brooks, and C. Love, 1993. "Breast cancer and silicone implants: Psychological consequences for women." *Journal of the National Cancer Institute* 85:1361–1365.

Hausner, R. J., F. J. Schoen, and K. K. Pierson. 1978. "Foreign-body reaction to silicone gel in auxillary lymph nodes after an augmentation mammoplasty." *Plastic and Reconstructive Surgery* 62:381–384.

Hennekens, C. H., I-Min Lee, N. Cook, P. Hebert, E. Karlson, F. LaMotte, J. Manson, and J. Buring. 1996. "Self-reported breast implants and connective-tissue diseases in female health professionals: A retrospective cohort study." *Journal of the American Medical Association* 275 8:616–621.

Hill, Sir A. B. 1965, January 14. "The environment and disease: Association or causation?" *Proceedings of the Royal Society of Medicine, Section of Occupational Medicine*. 9:295–300.

Hilts, P. 1992, January 13. "Maker of implants balked at tests, its records show." *New York Times*. pp. A.1, B.10.

Hochschild, A. 1989. *The Second Shift: Working Parents and Revolution at Home*. New York: Viking Press.

Hodgkinson, Darryl J. 1993. "The place for cosmetic surgery: Part 2. Body contouring." *Modern Medicine* 36:66.

Hopkins v. Dow Corning Corp., No. C-91–2132, 1991. U.S. Dist. LEXIS (N.D. Cal. May 27, 1992).

Hopkins v. Dow Corning Corp., 33F 3d 1116 (9th Dec. 1994).

Huber, Peter. 1991. *Galileo's Revenge: Junk Science in the Courtroom.* New York: Basic Books.

Ingersoll, B. 1992, January 13. "FDA review of Dow Corning documents led to call for moratorium on implants." *Wall Street Journal.* p. A.3.

Inlander, Charles B. 1993. "Medical hucksterism is still with us." *Nursing and Health Care* 14:313.

Jackson, L. A. 1992. *Physical Appearance and Gender: Sociobiological and Sociocultural Perspectives.* Albany, N.Y.: State University of New York Press.

Jaggar, A. M. and P. S. Rothenberg. 1993. *Feminist Frameworks.* New York: McGraw-Hill.

Japenga, A. 1993. "Face-lift city." *Health* 7 (2):46.

Jennings, N. R. v. Baxter Healthcare Corporation, A9405–03148, Vol. 16, Circuit Court of Oregon, December 5, 1995.

Jennings v. Baxter. 1995, December 5. 15:11. Proceedings.

Jenny, H. 1994. *Silicone-gate.* Siloam Springs, Ariz.: Henry Jenny.

Jensen, J. A., and M. J. Silverstein. 1993. "Doctor, should I have my breast implants removed?" *Emergency Medicine* 25:18.

Jones, J. H. 1993. *Bad Blood: The Tuskegee Syphilis Experiment.* New York: Free Press.

Kaslow, Florence and Hilton Becker. 1992. "Breast augmentation: Psychological and plastic surgery considerations." *Psychotherapy* 29:467–473.

Keithley-Johnston, K. 1997, October 23. Toxic discovery network: AOL communication.

Kessler, D. A. 1992. "The basis of the FDA's decision on breast implants." *New England Journal of Medicine* 326:1713–1715.

Kessler, D. A., R. B. Merkatz, and R. Schapiro, 1993. "A call for higher standards for breast implants." *Journal of the American Medical Association* 270:2607–2608.

Khan, S. S., S. Nessim, R. Gray, L. S. Czer, A. Chaux, and J. Matloff. 1990. "Increased mortality of women in coronary bypass surgery: Evidence in referral bias." *Annals of Internal Medicine* 112:561–567.

Kolata, Gina. 1996, February 28. "Study says implant risk, if any, is small: Both sides in legal battle say research vindicates their claims." *The New York Times.* p. 1.

Kolata, Gina. 1997, December 19. "Judge dismisses implant evidence." *The New York Times.* p. A1.

Kramer, R. 1984. "Corporate criminality: The development of an idea." In E. Hochstedler, ed., *Corporations as Criminals*, pp. 13–37. Beverly Hills, Calif.: Sage.

Krueger, D. W. 1990. "Developmental and psychodynamic perspectives on body image change." In T. F. Cash and D. Pruzinski, eds., *Body Images: Development, Deviance and Change.* New York: Guilford Press.

Lakoff, R., and R. Scherr, 1984. *Face Value: The Politics of Beauty.* New York: Routledge and Kegan Paul.

Las Vegas Sun, 1997, August 25. "Breast implant settlement offered." p. 1B.

Lawson, C. 1989, June 15. "Toys: Girls still apply makeup, boys fight wars." *The New York Times*. pp. C1, C10.

Lentz, A. J., M. L. Changler, and P. R. LeVier. 1978. *Biological Evaluation of an Implantable Silicone Gel: Summary of Acute and Chronic Studies*. Dow Corning document #154000246–154000266, exhibit to Weyenberg deposition.

Letvak, J. 1996, July 10. Letter to the editor. *Journal of the American Medical Association* 276 (2):102.

Levine, J. J., and N. T. Ilowite. 1994. "Scleroderma-like esophageal disease in children breast-fed by mothers with silicone breast implants." *Journal of the American Medical Association* 271:213–216.

Lindsey, Heidi et al. v. Dow Corning Corporation. CV-94-P-11558-S. Silicon Gel Breast Implants Products Liability Litigation MDL 926, March 29, 1994.

Loeske, D., and S. Cahill. 1984. "The social construction of deviance: Experts on battered women." *Social Problems* 31 (3):296–310.

Lofland, J., and R. Stark. 1965. "Becoming a world saver: A theory of conversion to a deviant perspective. *American Sociological Review* 30:862–875.

Lorde, Audre. 1980. *The Cancer Journals*. Argyle, N.Y.: Spinsters, Inc.

Lowe, Ben. 1994. "Body image and the politics of beauty: Foundations of the feminine ideal in medieval and early modern Europe." In K. Callaghan, ed., *Ideals of Feminine Beauty*, pp. 21–36. Westport, Conn.: Greenwood Press.

Lynch, W., W. Stith. 1980, April 14. Memo to field force. *Surgitec*. MEA (7056) 22–25.

MacKinnon, C. 1979. *Sexual Harassment of Working Women: A Case of Sex Discrimination*. New Haven: Yale University Press.

Mahlum, Charlotte and Marvin S. Mahlum v. Dow Chemical. CV 93–05941 Second Judicial District. Nevada, 1995.

Mahlum Memorandum, Factual Cite, *Mahlum v. Dow Chemical*, 1995.

Maugh II, Thomas H. 1996, February 28. "Implant study find little autoimmune disease risk." *Los Angeles Times*, p. 1:15.

Mazur, A. 1986. "U.S. trends in feminism, beauty and overadaptation." *Journal of Sex Research* 22:281–303.

McCarthy, E. J., R. B. Merkatz, and G. P. Bagley. 1993. "A descriptive analysis of physical complaints from women with silicone breast implants." *Journal of Women's Health* 2:111–115.

MDL-926 Silicone Breast Implant Litigation, Baxter 83650–83652.

MDL-926 Silicone Breast Implant Litigation, MCG 14431–14432.

MDL-926 Silicone Breast Implant Litigation, MMM 4960–4962.

Mead, G. H. 1934. *Mind, Self and Society*. Chicago: University of Chicago Press.

Mellemkjaer, L., J. K. McLaughlin, and J. F. Fraumeni, Jr. 1994. "Re: Breast implants, cancer, and systemic sclerosis." *Journal of the National Cancer Institute* 86:1424.

Merkatz, R. B., G. P. Bagley, and E. J. McCarthy. 1993. "A qualitative analysis of self-reported experiences among women encountering difficulties with silicone breast implants." *Journal of Women's Health* 2:105–109.

Merlin, Mildred v. 3M/McGhan. CVN 95–696HDM. U.S. District Court. 1996. Dist. of Nevada.

Meyrowitz, J. 1985. *No Sense of Place.* New York: Oxford University Press.

Miller, T. M., J. G. Coffman, and R. A. Linke. 1980. "Survey on body image: Weight and diet of college students." *Journal of the American Dietetic Association* 77:561–566.

Murphy, John. 1994. "Symbolic Violence and the Disembodiment of Identity." In K. Callaghan, ed., *Ideals of Feminine Beauty: Philosophical, Social, and Cultural Dimensions,* pp. 69–77. Westport, Conn.: Greenwood Press.

Noone, R. B. 1994, September 7, 9. Deposition MDL 926 Deposed by Scheller.

Onken, Henry D. 1994. "The impact of the media on women with breast implants." *Plastic and Reconstructive Surgery* 93:1312.

Pagelow, M. 1989. *Family Violence.* New York: Praeger.

Painter, Kim. 1996, February 28. "Implant study shows small autoimmune disease risk." *USA Today.* 2d.

Palcheff-Wiemer, M., M. Concannon, V. Conn, and C. Puckett. 1992. "The impact of media on women with breast implants." *Plastic and Reconstructive Surgery* 925:779–785.

Pardue, A. J. 1976, September 27. Letter to Don McGhan. McGhan Medical Corp.

Parker, Lisa. 1995. "Beauty and breast implantation: How candidate selection affects autonomy and informed consent." *Hypatia* 101:183–202.

Parks, T. 1996, December 23 and 30. "Fidelity." *The New Yorker,* pp. 54–60.

Pervitz, Kathrin. 1970. *Beyond the Looking Glass: America's Beauty Culture.* New York: William Morrow and Co.

Peters, W., E. Keystone, and D. Smith. 1994. "Factors affecting the rupture of silicon-gel breast implants." *Annals of Plastic Surgery* 32:449–451.

Pfuhl, E. H., and S. Henry. 1993. *The Deviance Process.* New York: Aldine.

Phillips, J. W., D. L. de Camara, M. D. Lockwood, and W. C. C. Grebner. 1996. "Strength of silicone breast implants." *Plastic and Reconstructive Surgery* 97:1215–1225.

Plaintiffs' response to defendants further memorandum on G. L. C. 93 A, post hearing developments on the issue of causation. Draft. 1996, December 27. C.A. 93: 5750. Middlesex, MA.

Plaintiffs' submission and proposed finding to the National Science Panel on silicone gel breast implants. 1997, October 6.

Plaintiffs' Trial Statement, Sec. 111, Statement of Undisputed Facts; Section 11, Causes of Action and Supporting Facts, Part E, Fraudulent Misrepresentation/Concealment. 1995, December 21. Mahlum v. Dow Chemical, CV 93–05941.

Plastic Reconstructive Surgery. 1976, March. 57:3. Heyer-Schuete Corporation Advertisement, "Our View . . . It Should Be Yours."

Plastic Reconstructive Surgery. 1988, March. 81:3. Dow Corning Wright Advertisement, "Mammary Implant with a Warranty."

Pollack, P. H. and M. E. Vittas. 1995. "Who bears the burdens of environmental pollution?: Race, ethnicity, and environmental equity in Florida." *Social Science Quarterly* 76 (2):294–310.

Pollitt, Katha. 1994. *Reasonable Creatures*. New York: Vintage.

Porterfield, H. W. 1982. "Comments on the proposal classification of inflatable prostheses." American Society of Plastic and Reconstructive Surgeons. Chicago, Illinois.

Porterfield, W. 1983. "The challenges for plastic surgeons." *Plastic and Reconstructive Surgery* 71 (5)703–705.

Press, R. I., C. L. Peebles, Y. Kuma, R. L. Ochs, and E. M. Tan. 1992. "Antinuclear autoantibodies in women with silicone breast implants." *The Lancet* 340: 1304–1307.

Randall, Teri. 1992a. "Antibodies to silicone detected in patients with severe inflammatory reactions." *Journal of the American Medical Association* 268:1821.

Randall, Teri. 1992b. "Surgeons grapple with synovitis, fractures around silicone implants for hand and wrist." *Journal of the American Medical Association* 268:13.

Regush, Nicholas. 1992, January/February. "Toxic breasts." *Mother Jones*, pp. 24–31.

Reissman, C. K. 1983. "Women and medicalization: A new perspective." *Social Policy* 14:3–18.

Renzetti, C. M., and D. J. Curran. 1992. *Women, Men, and Society*. Boston: Allyn and Bacon.

Rheingold, H. L., and K. V. Cook. 1975. "The contents of boys' and girls' rooms as an index of parents' behaviors." *Child Development* 46:459–463.

Richardson, L., and V. Taylor. 1993. *Feminist Frontiers 111*. New York: McGraw-Hill.

Robbins, J. 1996. *Reclaiming Your Health*. Tiburon, Calif.: H.L. Kramer Publishing Co.

Robinson, Jr., O. G., E. L. Bradley, and D. S. Wilson. 1995. "Analysis of explanted silicone implants: A report of 300 patients." *Annals of Plastic Surgery* 34:1–7.

Roiphe, K. 1993. *The Morning After: Sex, Fear, and Feminism on Campus*. Boston: Little, Brown.

Rowe, V. K, et al. 1948. "Toxicological studies on certain commercial silicone and hydrolyzable saline intermediates." *Journal of Industrial Hygiene and Toxicology* 30:332–352.

Rowland, J., J. Holland, T. Changlassian, and D. Kinne. 1993. "Psychological response to breast reconstruction." *Psychosomatics* 343:241–250.

Russell, D. 1982. *Rape in Marriage*. New York: Macmillan.

Rynbrant, L. J., and R. C. Kramer. 1995. "Hybrid nonwomen and corporate violence: The silicone breast implant case." *Violence Against Women* 1:206–227.

Saduak, J. 1965, June 28. FDA letter to P. Schneider re: Silicone fluids. DCCKMM (280) 3804–3805.

Sahn, E. E., P. D. Garen, R. M. Silver, and J. C. Maize. 1990. "Scleroderma following augmentation mammoplasty: Report of a case and review of the literature." *Archives of Dermatology* 126:1198–1201.

Sanchez-Guerrero, J., G. A. Colditz, E. W. Karlson, D. J. Hunter, F. E. Speizer, and M. H. Liang. 1995. "Silicone breast implants and the risk of connective-tissue diseases and symptoms." *New England Journal of Medicine* 332:1666–1669.

Sanchez-Guerrero, J., P. H. Schur, J. S. Sergent, and M. H. Laing. 1994. "Silicone breast implants and rheumatic disease: Clinical, immunologic, and epidemiologic studies." *Arthritis and Rheumatism* 37(2):158.

Schaef, A. 1987. *When Society Becomes an Addict.* San Francisco: Harper and Row.

Schilder, P. 1950. *The Image and Appearance of the Human Body.* New York: International University Press.

Schmitt, R. B. 1996, December 19. "Women in silicone cases suffer big setback." *The Wall Street Journal.* p. B8.

Schumann, Delores. 1994. "Health risks for women with breast implants." *The Nurse Practitioner* 19:19.

Schur, Edwin. 1984. *Labeling Women Deviant.* New York: Random House.

Schusterman, M. A., S. S. Kroll, G. P. Reece, et al. 1993. "Evidence of autoimmune disease in patients after breast reconstruction with silicone gel implants versus autogenous tissue: A preliminary report." *Annals of Plastic Surgery* 31:1–6.

Scully, D. and J. Marolla, 1993. "Convicted rapists' vocabulary of motives: Excuses and justifications." In D. Kelly, ed., *Deviant Behavior.* New York: St. Martin's Press.

Sheller, Stephen A. 1995. "Will the real junk science please stand up: An analysis of the May Clinic Women's Study and Harvard/Brigham Nurses Study in relation to the silicone gel breast implant controversy." *Mealey's Litigation Report: Breast Implants* IV(1):1–8.

Shiffman, Melvin A. 1994. "Silicone breast implant litigation Part 1." *Medicine and Law* 13:681–716.

Shiffman, Melvin A. 1995. "Silicone breast implant litigation Part 2." *Medicine and Law* 14:59–85.

Silver, M., E. E. Sahn, J. A. Allen, S. Sahn, W. Greene, J. C. Maize, et al. 1993. "Demonstration of silicone in sites of connective-tissue disease in patients with silicone-gel breast implants." *Archives of Dermatology* 129:63–68.

Silverman, B., S. L. Brown, R. Bright, R. Kaczmarek, J. Arrowsmith-Lowe, and D. Kessler, 1996. "Reported complications of silicone gel breast implants: an epidemiologic review." *Annals of Internal Medicine* 1248:744–755.

Simon, Michele. 1995. "The silicone gel breast implant controversy: The science surrounding the regulation and litigation." *Journal of Products & Toxics Liability* 17:141–162.

Skogerson, K. E. 1995, December 11. "Dow Chemical case: Judge obviously biased [Letter to the editor]." *Reno Gazette Journal*, p. 11A.

Spector, M., and J. Kitsuse, 1977. *Constructing Social Problems*, Menlo Park, Calif.: Benjamin Cummings Publishing Co.

Speira, Harry. 1988. "Scleroderma after silicone augmentation mammoplasty." *Journal of the American Medical Association* 2:236.

Spitzack, C. 1990. *Confessing Excess: Women and the Politics of Body Reduction.* Albany, N.Y.: State University of New York Press.

Stauber, John C., and Sheldon Rampton. 1996. "Science under pressure: Dow-funded studies say "no problem." *PR Watch: Public Interest Reporting on the PR/Public Affairs Industry* 4(1): first quarter.

Steinmetz, S., M. Strauss, and R. Gelles. 1980. *Behind Closed Doors*. Garden City, N.Y.: Anchor Books.

Stern v. Dow Corning Corp. 83–2348, 1984.

Stewart, M. 1997. "Judicature." Review of *Science on Trial*, M. Angell, 1996.

Stewart, M. 1992. *Gender Bias in Sexual Assault Cases: A Study of the Nevada Justice System*. Report for the Nevada Supreme Court Task Force on Gender Bias.

Stewart, M. 1991. "The redefinition of incest: From sin to sickness." *Family Science* 4(1–2):53–68.

Stewart, M., and J. Ross. 1996. "Discreditable stigma: The intersection of femininity and plastic surgery." Pacific Sociological Association meetings, Seattle.

Stewart, M., S. Dobbin, and S. Gatowski. 1996, August. "A study of shared definitions of reality in rape cases." *Feminist Legal Studies*. Vol. IV, no. 2. pp. 159–177.

Stombler, Robin E. 1993. "Breast implants and the FDA: Past, present, and future." *Bulletin of the American College of Surgeons* 78:11.

Strauss, M. A., and R. J. Gelles. 1990. *Physical Violence in American Families: Risk Factors and Adaptions to Violence in 8,145 Families*. New Brunswick, N.J.: Transaction.

Subby, R., and J. Friel. 1984. *Co-dependency and family rules*. Pompano Beach, Fla.: Health Communications, Inc.

Sullivan, Deborah. 1993. Cosmetic surgery: Market dynamics and medicalization. *Research in the Sociology of Health Care* 19: 97–115.

Taubes, Gary. 1995, December. "Silicone in the system." *Discover*, 65–75.

Thompson, J. K., L. A. Penner, and M. N. Altabe. 1990. "Procedures, problems and progress in the assessment of body images." In T. F. Cash and D. Pruzinski, eds., *Body Images: Development, Deviance and Change*. New York: Guilford Press.

Thompson, J. K., and S. Tantleff. 1992. "Female and male ratings of upper torso: Actual, ideal, and stereotypical conceptions." *Journal of Social Behavior and Personality* 7:345–354.

Tiemersma, D. 1989. *Body Schema and Body Image*. Amsterdam: Swets and Zeitlinger.

Tseëlon, Efrat. 1995. *The Masque of Femininity: The Presentation of Woman in Everyday Life*. Thousand Oaks, Calif.: Sage Publications.

Unger, R. 1985. "Personal appearance and social control." In M. Safir, M. Mednick, D. Izraeli, and J. Bernard, eds., *Women's Worlds: The New Scholarship*. New York: Praeger.

U.S. Congress, House of Representatives. 1993. *The FDA's Regulation of Silicone Breast Implants*. Committee on Government Operations. 102nd session. Washington, D.C.: U.S. Government Printing Office.

U.S. Food and Drug Administration. 1993. *Breast Implants: A Consumer Information Update*. Rockville, Md.

Valentine, Catherine. 1994. "Female bodily perfection and the divided self." *Ideals of Feminine Beauty: Philosophical, Social, and Cultural Dimensions*. Westport, Conn.: Greenwood Press.

Van Nunen, S. A., P. A. Gelenby, and A. Basten. 1982. "Postmammoplasty connective tissue disease." *Arthritis and Rheumatology* 25:694–697.

Van Voris, B. 1997, November 24. "Implants suits to proceed in Michigan court." *National Law Journal*. p. B.1.

Varga, J., H. R. Schumacher, and S. A. Jimenez. 1989. "Systemic sclerosis after augmentation mammoplasty with silicone implants." *Annals of Internal Medicine* 3:377–383.

Vasey, F., and J. Feldstein. 1993. *The Silicone Breast Implant Controversy*. Freedom, Calif.: Crossing Press.

Walker, L., and J. Monahan. 1996. "Daubert and the Reference Manual: An essay on the future of science in law." *Virginia Law Review* 82:5.

Wallen, J. 1979. "Physician stereotypes about female health and illness." *Women and Health* 4:135–46.

Wall Street Journal, 1995, November 8. "Review and outlook: Junk science and judges." p. A18.

Washburn, J. 1996, March/April. "Reality check: Can 400,000 women be wrong?" *Ms.*, 51–57.

Washington Post, 1996, December 18. "Sickness and science in the court." p. C6.

Wegscheider-Cruse S. 1981. *Another Chance: Hope and Health for the Alcoholic Family*. Palo Alto, Calif.: Science and Behavior Books.

Weisman, M. H., T. R. Vecchione, D. Albert, L. T. Moore, and M. R. Mueller. 1988. "Connective-tissue disease following breast augmentation: A preliminary test of the human adjuvant disease hypothesis." *Journal of Plastic, Reconstructive Surgery* 82:626–630.

Weitzman, L. 1974. *Sex Role Socialization: A Focus on Women*. Palo Alto, Calif.: Mayfield.

Weitzman, L. 1985. *The Divorce Revolution*. New York: Free Press.

Weitzman, L. 1988. "Women and children last: The social and economic consequences of divorce law reforms." In S. Dornbusch and M. Strober, eds., *Feminism, Children, and the New Families*. New York: Guilford Press.

Wells, K. E., C. W. Cruse, and J. L. Baker. 1994. "The health status of women following cosmetic surgery." *Plastic and Reconstructive Surgery* 93:907–912.

West, C., and D. Zimmerman. 1987. "Doing gender." *Gender & Society* 1:125–151.

White, G. 1996, October. Personal communication.

Winer, E., K. Fee-Fulkerson, C. Fulkerson, G. Georgaide, K. Catoe, M. Conaway, V. H. Brunatti, and B. Rimer. 1993. "Silicone controversy: A survey of women with breast cancer and silicone implants." *Journal of the National Cancer Institute* 8517:1407–1411.

Woititz, J. 1983. *Adult Children of Alcoholics*. Pompano Beach, Fla.: Health Communications.

Wolf, N. 1991. *The Beauty Myth: How Images of Beauty Are Used Against Women*. New York: William Morrow.

Wood, Julia. 1994. *Gendered Lives: Communication, Gender, and Culture*. Belmont, Calif.: Wadsworth Publishing Co.

Yoshida, S. H., C. C. Chang, S. S. Teuber, and M. E. Gershwin. 1993. "Silicon and silicone: Theoretical and clinical implications of breast implants." *Regulatory Toxicology and Pharmacology* 17:3–18.

Yu, L. T., G. Latorre, J. Marotta, C. Batich, and N. S. Hardt. 1996. "In vitro measurement of silicone bleed from breast implants." *Plastic and Reconstructive Surgery* 97:756–763.

Zones, J. S. 1992. "The political and social context of silicone breast implant use in the United States." *Journal of Long-Term Effects of Medical Implants* 1:225–241.

Index

Self-esteem, 51, 56, 64, 74, 80, 93, 95, 103, 123

Sexual harrassment, 185

Side effects. *See* Complications; Diseases, systemic; Symptoms of implant related disease

Silica, 28

Silicone: inertness, 8, 28, 29, 32, 36, 38, 45, 153, 162, 202; injections, 17, 27, 29, 31, 36, 45; leakage, 8, 18, 19, 31–33, 40–45, 100–09, 153, 154, 161; liquid, 8, 17, 18, 27, 28, 29, 32, 35, 36

Silverman, Stuart, Dr., 26, 163

Simon, Michele, 17, 19, 27

Sjögren's Syndrome, 44, 104, 105

Small breasts, as deformities and disease, 9, 51, 76, 79, 91, 94, 103, 121, 122

Social construction: of reality, 128, 129, 162, 190; of medical records, 129, 132–33, 141, 143

Spector, Malcolm, Judge, 193

Spokin, Stanley, Judge, 41

Steinheimer, Connie, Judge, 159, 180

Stern, Maria, 2, 187

Stigma: 63, 79, 91, 99, 100, 122, 123; advocates, 119–21; path, 115–99; preventing 124–25; restimagtizing, 121–24

Surgical entrepreneur, 68

Surgitek Company, 31, 44, 45, 47, 48, 50

Symptoms of implant related disease: aches and pains, 94, 103, 104, 108, 110, 123, 130; arthralgia, 105; bladder infection, 113; depression, 20, 97, 98, 130, 138, 163; dizziness, 138; esophageal immotility, 40, definition, 201; fatigue, 40, 94, 104, 105, 108, 112, 113, 123, 130, 138; fever, 94, 105, 113; flu-like symptoms, 40, 94, 103, 110; hair loss, 18, 40, 105, 108, 123; headaches, 40, 94, 109, 110, 123, 138; hematoma, 171; inflammation, 5, 35, 47, 171, itching, 108–10; joint pain, 93, 105, 138; memory loss, 18, 40, 93, 104, 108, 123; muscle pain, 44, 105; neurological disorders, 40, 113; night sweats, 20, 138, 153; Raynaud's, 18, 40, 105, 110; sleeplessness, 20, 108, 110, 130

"Theory of the office," 135

Toluenediamine (TDA), 31, 34, 48, 203

Tort reform, 2, 5, 11, 19, 85, 159

Toxic dumps, 18, 192–96

U. S. House Subcommittee on Government Affairs (U.S. Congress, 1993), 10, 17, 26, 35, 38, 41, 43–52

Vasallo v. Baxter, 160

Victim: blaming the, 86, 87, 187; of harassment, 188; of rape, 188; "real," 186

Victimization, 64, 74

Violence: against women, 51, 184, 185; battery and, 74, 184, 186, 190, 194; breast implants as, 184, 186, 187; experts' response, 189, 191; harassment and, 184, 185, 186, 190, 194; long-term impact, 141, 194, 195; rape and, 184, 186, 190, 194; self-blame and, 188; social construction of, 184–86; subsequent behavior and, 188

Weiss, Ted, Congressman, 26, 42, 43, 183

White, Geoff, 108, 177

Y-ME, 18, 26, 47

About the Author

MARY WHITE STEWART is Associate Professor of Sociology and Director of the Interdisciplinary Ph.D. Program at the University of Nevada, Reno. She teaches and writes in the areas of gender, family violence, social psychology, and deviance. She was the jury consultant for the plaintiff in the *Mahlum v. Dow Chemical* case.